This book is de

T O U C H I N

Touch me ,

Touch me , to show that we are here .

Touch me , to show that you can help .

Touch me , but not too much .

Touching is not learned ,

Not touching is .

J Byrom

IV

CONTENTS

			Page
Section 1	-	Clinical Placement	1
Section 2	-	Anthropometry	19
Section 3	-	Nutritional Requirements	29
Section 4	-	Enteral Nutrition	45
Section 5	-	Parenteral Nutrition	61
Section 6	-	Drugs	69
Section 7	-	Product Information	79
Section 8	-	General Data	105

TABLES

Page

Section 1

1.1 Example of a clinical placement time table   3

Section 2

2.1 Height conversion table   21
2.2 Weight conversion table   22
2.3 Grades of obesity (BMI)   23
2.4 Desirable weight/height in adults (men)   24
2.5 Desirable weight/height in adults (women)   25
2.6 Desirable weight/height in children   26
2.7 Average weight gain in infancy   27

Section 3

3.1 Approximate guide to estimating BMR   29
3.2 Schofield equation   29
3.3 Harris-Benedict equation   30
3.4 PENG guidelines for general adult
     nutritional requirements   32
3.5 Adult Estimated Average Requirements
     for energy   34
3.6 Adult Reference Nutrient Intakes for protein   35
3.7 Adult Dietary Reference Values for fat and
     carbohydrate   36

3.8   Adult Reference Nutrient Intakes for vitamins   37
3.9   Adult Reference Nutrient Intakes for minerals
      (SI Units)   38
3.10 Adult Reference Nutrient Intakes for
      minerals (mg/d)   39
3.11 Adult safe intakes for vitamins and minerals   40
3.12 Paediatric selected dietary Reference
      Nutrient Intakes   41

Section 4

4.1   Complications associated with tube feeding   54

Section 6

6.1   Oral hypoglycaemics   70
6.2   Common insulins   71
6.3   Common drugs used in the treatment of acute
      and chronic diarrhoea   72
6.4   Drugs which may cause diarrhoea   73
6.5   Drugs used to relieve constipation   74
6.6   Drugs that can cause constipation   74
6.7   Common drug examples of diuretics   75
6.8   Lipid lowering drugs   75
6.9   Drug-nutrient interactions   76
6.10 Common drug examples of antiemetics   77
6.11 Common drug examples of appetite
      stimulants and suppressants   77

Section 7

7.1   Sip feeds (milk based)   82
7.2   Sip feeds (fruit flavoured)   85
7.3   Tube feeds (whole protein)   87
7.4   Tube feeds (elemental and semi-elemental)   92
7.5   Fortified milk shakes (powders)   94
7.6   Fortified puddings   96
7.7   Fortified soups   97

		Page
7.8	Energy supplements	98
7.9	Protein supplements	101
7.10	Thickeners	102

Section 8

8.1	Useful conversion factors	105
8.2	Clinical blood biochemistry reference ranges	106
8.3	Medical shorthand	109
	Medical abbreviations	110
	Useful diet history/food abbreviations	118
8.4	Food portion sizes and weights 'common foods'	120
8.5	Nutritional composition of hospital food	121
8.6	Nutritional composition of 'common foods'	122
8.7	Energy content of alcoholic beverages	123
	Recommended alcohol intakes	124
8.8	Weaning Guide	125
8.9	Water soluble vitamins	128
8.10	Fat soluble vitamins	129
8.11	Minerals	130
8.12	Chemical elements and symbols	131
8.13	A guide to religious influences on diet	132
8.14	Nutrient absorption sites in the Gastro-intestinal tract	135
8.15	Amino acids in man	136
8.16	Normal fluid balance (adults)	136
8.17	Dietetic and nutrition internet sites	137
8.18	UK manufacturers' addresses for clinical nutrition products	138
8.19	Dietetic addresses - other	142

FIGURES

Page

Section 2
2.1   Anthropometric sites   20

Section 3
3.1   Elia Normagram   31

Section 4
4.1   Administration and indications for tube
      or parenteral feeding   46
4.2   Example routes of administration - short term   48
4.3   Example routes of administration - long term   49
4.4   Example of a 1500kcal Naso-Gastric pump
      starter feeding regimen   55
4.5   Example of a 2000kcal Naso-Gastric pump
      starter feeding regimen   56

Section 5
5.1   Parenteral nutrition - routes of administration   62

Section 8
8.1   Anatomy of the Gastro-intestinal tract   134

CONTRIBUTORS

ZOE JENKINS, SRD
St. James Hospital, Leeds

ANITA UPRICHARD, SRD
North Tyneside General Hospital

ACKNOWLEDGEMENTS

Thank you to everyone involved in turning this book from an idea in to a reality. In particular, to the Queen Margaret College Dietetic Students (Year 1992 - 1996) who helped with the essential background research of this book; to all the dietitians who expressed an interest and gave constructive comments and content ideas; to all those who have helped with proof reading; to my family and friends; to all the Nutrition Companies who helped financially support this project. Finally, and specifically, my thanks to:

THE ROYAL BOURNEMOUTH HOSPITAL DIETETIC DEPARTMENT

FIONA MURRAY
Publishing Consultant, Edinburgh

SUE HARVEY
Medical Staff Committee Office
The Royal Bournemouth Hospital

DR RICHARD DUNNILL
Consultant Anaesthetist
The Royal Bournemouth Hospital

JACQUI BOWDEN
Senior Pharmacist
The Royal Bournemouth Hospital

DR NICHOLAS HERODOTOU
Senior House Officer
The Royal Bournemouth Hospital

FINANCIAL ASSISTANCE FROM

Fresenius Ltd
H J Heinz Co Ltd
Kimal Pharmaceutical Products
Nestlé Clinical Nutrition
Nestlé UK Ltd
Nutricia Clinical Care
Ross Products, A Division of Abbott
Sutherland Health
Scientific Hospital Supplies
The Royal Bournemouth and Christchurch Hospitals NHS Trust
Unigreg Ltd

PREFACE

Accurate and well-referenced material is vital to all Dietitians. This handy compendium is an excellent source of valuable information for students and State Registered Dietitians alike. It will replace that large, indispensable but rather unwieldy bundle of dog-eared, folded pieces of paper found in the pocket of a white coat, or carried precariously in a filofax or kardex. Keeping up-to-date is one of the cornerstones of continuing professional development thus making the 'Dietitian's Pocket Book' a useful addition to any Dietitian's library, provided it does not just sit on the shelf.

The British Dietetic Association's strategy is to ensure that the whole profession practises continuing professional development. Joining The British Dietetic Association will help facilitate this, now and in the future.

Isabel Skypala
Honorary Education Officer
The British Dietetic Association

A note from the Author

Dear Reader

Through my recent experience as a dietetic student at The Royal London Hospital, I realised that there was a lack of reference pocket books available specifically for UK student dietitians on clinical placement. Consequently I spent my final year honours project researching what the dietetics world would like to see in this book.

It is aimed specifically at student dietitians on clinical placement but it contains general data which I hope many dietitians and health care professionals will also find useful. As I'm sure you'll appreciate, with the many differences in hospital reference ranges, protocols and not least student training, it is impossible to produce a data book specifically suited to every individual. I do, however, hope that this book goes some way to cover what is currently lacking.

Comments, contributions and suggestions for future editions are most welcome (c/o Amino Acid Books). Meanwhile, to those of you still training, all the very best and good luck!

Ms. Sarah Byrom
BSc (Hons), SRD

Using the book - Notes

General

- This book is intended as a reference guide only. In all cases, reference ranges specific to individual hospitals must be used as appropriate
- Examples of clinical and dietetic procedures are also given as a guide. These will vary from hospital to hospital, therefore always refer to your own hospital's training time table, standards, procedures and protocols
- For continual up-to-date information always consult current information
- Medical and Dietetic abbreviations are used throughout the book. The following reference pages will list most of these in full:

Abbreviations	**Page**
Medical	110
Diet History	118
Chemical Elements	131

Section 1

- This section is primarily based on my own experience as a dietetic student on clinical placement only. Students should therefore always refer to the specific standards and procedures of the hospital in which they work
- The actual time structure of clinical placement will be changing. It is intended that clinical placement will be more spread out over the time of studying rather than the current 31 week block
- The taking of a diet history referred to in this section has been outlined very simplistically, it is based on an in-patient having three set meals a day. In practise this will vary tremendously, according to the individual, and should be adapted accordingly
- The system of patient hospital admissions will vary from hospital to hospital

Section 2

- Very basic examples of anthropometry have been described in this section. For further details the reader should refer to references under 'further reading' at the end of this section

Section 3

- Examples of calculating a patient's 'general' nutritional requirements are outlined. The reader should refer elsewhere for calculating the nutritional requirements of speciality dietetic patients, eg paediatrics, nutritional support etc

Sections 4 and 5

- A very general overview of nutritional support has been given in these two sections. Although students will be actively involved with enteral nutrition this will almost always be less so than for parenteral nutrition, as the latter requires even more specialist dietetic knowledge and experience

Section 6

- For current drug information always consult an up-to-date BNF, MIMS or a Pharmacist

Section 7

- Always consult company product information services/ literature and the BNF/MIMS for up-to-date product information
- Speciality feeds, eg those for paediatrics and metabolic disorders, are not included in this section
- Blank tables have been included in this section to add up-to-date product information and/or new nutritional products

Section 8

- Lists useful, general data
- Biochemical references ranges and dietetic abbreviations will vary from hospital to hospital

Section 1

Clinical Placement

Introduction

Pre-placement

- The current UK Clinical training for an undergraduate dietitian is 28 weeks in all over a 31 week period. As a guide, 24 weeks of this time will be spent at a base-trainer hospital (ie main hospital), five weeks at a complementary hospital and two weeks holiday

- Prior to placement, you will receive information on all base-trainer hospitals to decide which one you would like to go to. Complementary placement is normally decided on during the early weeks of clinical placement

- Choosing a base-trainer is a very individual choice but ultimately depends on the availability of student placements that a base-trainer can provide

- If you are unsure about which base-trainer to choose, speak to your course tutor or the clinical placement organiser

- Every effort is made to place students as fairly as possible, but certain students may need to be given special priority, eg those with children. In this instance, second and third base-trainer preferences must be considered

- Approximately 2 - 3 months prior to placement your base-trainer will send you general information regarding the hospital and accommodation (if applicable). Not all base-trainers will be able to provide hospital accommodation. Ensure you establish this with your base-trainer well before you begin your placement

- Financial allowances may be allocated for some clinical placements. These tend to be very small and payable only at the end of placement. Where applicable, consult your course tutor for current rates

- Some base-trainers may schedule your two week holiday within your time table before you commence placement. If you have already booked a holiday, ensure you inform your base-trainer of this in good time

During placement

- The aim of clinical placement is to train the student to a level whereby they are competent and capable of managing general inpatient and outpatient work unsupervised

- The workload involved would be that which is expected of a newly qualified dietitian and regularly reporting back to the appropriate dietitian would be expected

- Commonly seen patients, seen by basic grade dietitians, would include: malnourished, diabetic, obese, lipid lowering and enterally tube fed patients

- Clinical placement will also provide an overview of various dietetic specialities eg paediatrics, burns, renal etc

- Most base-trainers will arrange similar, time tables to the one in Table 1.1, adapted to the student's development(s), interests, hospital specialities and trainers available

- Half a day per week private study time should be allocated within your time table

- Each dietitian will comment on your progress on a weekly basis. You will also be able to discuss how you think you've progressed or perhaps what you may need extra help with

- Identify who your base-trainer student mentor is so you know who to liaise with should you have any queries/ problems during placement

- Approximately half way through clinical placement a course tutor from your academic institute will visit you and your base-trainer, to review your progress

- During the last four weeks of clinical placement you will be responsible for various wards and outpatient clinic(s) unsupervised, but reporting back regularly to the appropriate dietitian(s)

Table 1.1 - Example of a clinical placement time table

Week	Activity
1	Department induction. Familiarisation with hospital layout, office and catering procedures
2	Ward week. Shadow nurses on specific ward. Familiarisation with staff gradings and ward procedures
3 - 8	Shadowing Dietitian(s) for general dietetic in and outpatients. Including obese, diabetic, malnourished and tube fed patients. Begin to interview patients, take diet histories, document in medical/dietetic and nurses records (supervised). Assignment of individual tasks, eg computer dietary analyses, 'mini case studies' etc
9 - 11	Shadow Senior Dietitian, eg Renal, Community, Paediatrics, Liver, Diabetes. Begin main case study
12 - 13	Shadow Senior Dietitian
14 - 16	Two week holiday
17 - 22	Complementary Placement, consolidate existing knowledge of general dietetic patients. Expand on area(s) of interest
23 - 26	Specialist Dietitian(s) (Shadow). Study days, eg specialist dietetic depts in surrounding area, talks, lectures etc
27 - 31	4 weeks ward and out-patient management. Unaccompanied, but regularly reporting back to responsible dietitian(s). Main case study completed. Final appraisal and assessment

Example of dietetic referral procedures - inpatients (I/P)

Referral new inpatient - Checklist of procedures

- Check dietetic referral in medical notes or on a referral form (unethical to see patient otherwise, although some wards, eg ITU, may use a 'blanket' referral scheme)
- Read through medical notes
- Fill in relevant details on dietetic cards (eg patient's home address, GP, past medical history, present condition, social history, biochemistry and reason for dietetic referral)
- Speak to appropriate medical staff looking after patient (if required)
- Fill in bed-end folder details onto dietetic cards (eg present weight, height, bowel movements, temperature, fluid balance, medication, blood sugars, nutritional supplements and nasogastric feeding regimens, if applicable)
- Speak to patient and record information (introduce yourself and ask the patient if they know why they have been referred to a dietitian)
- Add relevant dietetic information to bed-end folder/nursing records (eg summary of assessment aims, nasogastric feeding regimen, meal plans, food intake charts and or special dietary instructions for medical staff to follow)
- Write dietary assessment and recommendations/aims in medical notes/nursing records
- Speak to nurse looking after patient, informing them of advice you have given to the patient
- Follow up as required, depending on the individual requirements of the patient and hospital dietetic review protocols

Time allowance

- To carry out above procedures usually between 30 - 40 minutes per new inpatient.
- Actual time spent will depend on available time and type of patient

Follow up inpatient - Checklist

- Check medical records
- "Hello (patient's name) how are you today?"
- "How have you been getting on with your food?" (or specify progress with previous dietary problems/aims discussed)
- Quick diet history (if necessary/time permits)
- Deal with any queries the patient may have and/or set new goals
- Inform patient when you will see them next
- Conclude interview

Time allowance

15 - 20 minutes.

General considerations

- Ensure you keep up-to-date with recent developments of your patient ie by checking medical notes and speaking to medical staff
- Document all follow-ups briefly in the dietetic cards and medical notes
- Record appropriate details (eg weight changes) in dietetic, medical and/or nursing records

Outpatients (O/P) - An overview

- Once patients are discharged from hospital, they will be followed up, where appropriate, eg in O/P clinics. Alternatively patients may be referred to dietetic O/P clinics via their GP or Consultant
- Follow the similar procedures and considerations outlined for I/P procedures. If you are seeing a new O/P, try to fill out their dietetic details on the dietetic records before seeing them, ie try to obtain medical notes pre-clinic

- If a new O/P is referred via their GP, normally a letter briefly outlining dietetic assessment details and advice is sent to the GP after the clinic by the dietitian

- Letters will also be sent to GPs if a patient fails to attend an appointment or is dishcharged from dietetic care

- Finding dietetic cards before the clinic starts will save time

- If medical notes are present, a very brief outline of dietetic advice/recommendations should be documented

- Above all, find out what O/P procedures your hospital has and follow them

Time allowance

20 - 30 minutes new O/P, 10 - 15 minutes follow up

Dietetic interview (new patient) - Checklist of content

- Introduce self - recap where referral is from

- Explain what you are going to do in the interview

- Identify problem - ensure that your perception of the problem is the same as the patients

- Establish height

- Establish current weight and BMI

- Weight history

- Diet history

- Advice to patient - agree on dietary goals that are set

- Patient has any questions?

- Review appointment arranged

- End interview

Diet History (24 hours) - Interview content (new inpatient)

1. **Introduce self**
   - "Hello my name is Jane Smith, I'm a student dietitian. Did the doctor/nurse/dietitian tell you I was coming to see you?" **or**
   - "Hello my name is Jane Smith, I'm a student dietitian. How have you been getting on with your food?" **or**
   - "Hi, my name is Jane Smith, I'm a student dietitian. I hear (or understand) you've been having problems with ....."

2. **Explain to patient the structure of interview**
   - Explain how you are going to ask them briefly about their weight history and food intake, then give them some dietary advice

3. **Patient's weight history - Ask the patient:**
   - Do they know how tall they are?
   - Do they know what weight they are? (to establish BMI)
   - Have they always been this weight?
   - How long has it taken them to have gained/lost this weight?

4. **Diet history (24 hour recall) - Ask the patient:**
   - What was the first thing you had to eat/drink?
   - Did you have any thing before lunch?
   - What did you have for lunch?
   - Did you have any thing before your evening meal?
   - What did you have for your evening meal?
   - Did you have any thing mid evening/before going to bed?
   - Did you eat any thing friends/relatives brought in?
   - Have you had any nutritional supplements (or 'special' drinks) from the nurses or other ward staff?
   - Have you had anything from the hospital shop and/or trolley?

NB The above (point 4) assumes the patient has regular meal times. For a more open, unassuming approach, try asking the patient what they ate next instead of using set meal times

5. **Summary and plan of action**
   - Summarise information gathered to the patient
   - Adapt and explain to patient meal plan/dietary advice
   - If applicable, let patient try nutritional supplements (to distinguish preferences)
   - Ask patient if they have any questions
   - Inform patient when they will see you again
   - Conclude interview

During diet history try to establish:
   - Quantities of food eaten, ask the patient if they ate all of their food and, if not, how much, or if they were sick/had diarrhoea, or why they did not eat all of their food. This will help to estimate the patient's current energy/protein intake
   - Fat/refined sugar content of food/drinks eaten, eg if a patient drinks milk is it full fat, semi-skimmed or skimmed?
   - Eating/digestive problems (eg swallowing)
   - Specific foods (if any) causing problems
   - Food preferences
   - Current carers (if any) able to bring food in

Diet History (24 hours) general considerations

- Although the previous section outlines the structure of seeing a patient, it is rare that this sequence of events occurs exactly in this order. However, as long as you introduce yourself and cover all essential points/areas then this doesn't matter too much

- What you look for in a patient's diet history depends on the type of patient. For example, with diabetics you would be looking especially for the total intake of simple sugars, fatty foods and complex carbohydrates; with malnourished patients you would be looking at intake of high energy protein foods and so on

- If patients 'ramble' at great length, or the interview is well over time, try rounding off advice as quickly as possible and stand up!

- Tests, Nil By Mouth etc may mean that the patient hasn't eaten anything for a while. Try to establish how long it is since they have eaten, as well as a typical food intake when eating 'normally'

- Some patients, especially chemotherapy patients, will have very irregular eating patterns, try to establish what they manage to eat on 'good' and 'bad' days

- Be aware of the side effects of certain medications which could cause nausea, vomiting and diarrhoea etc (refer to section 6)

- Always establish with the nurses/doctors how much a patient knows about their medical condition. Sometimes carers may know the diagnosis whereas some patients may be about to be told or choose not to know

- Patients may not always be there when you go to see them. If a patient is away for tests or treatment try to arrange a better time with the nurse or another time to see them

- Be aware of a patients physical/emotional state. If you feel it is inappropriate to see them or continue the interview, arrange to see them another time

- Treat each patient as an individual and explain to them what you're going to do (this will help to put the patient at ease)

- Avoid jargon. One way to assess if a patient has understood you is to ask them to restate what advice you have given them to follow

- Listen to a patient and try to be as empathetic and under-standing as possible. Avoid writing excessive notes during a patient interview, this may be off-putting for the patient as they may feel you are not listening properly to them

- Finally, if a patient has had no bowel movement for a considerable time, check the patient's food intake before recommending laxatives to nurses. You may find there is nothing inside the patient to cause a bowel movement in the first place or the patient is not hungry because they are constipated!

Hospital Catering Systems - An overview

- Hospital menus commonly follow a two to three week cycle
- Some hospital catering departments will have a diet bay or diet cook that can prepare special menus (such as adding protein/energy supplements or artificial sweeteners to foods)
- Meals may be served on the ward level, either by using a hot plate or individually trayed and portion controlled system
- Depending on budget holders, nutritional supplements may be stored at ward level, within the catering department, pharmacy and/or the dietetic department
- The patient's charter states that no patient should have to order more than one day's meals in advance and that ethnic menus should be available

Ward information - An overview

The Medical Team - Doctors
House Officers (HO's)

- These are newly qualified doctors (called 'pre-registration doctors') who begin work on the wards as their first appointments. They work for a specific Consultant and are supervised by a Senior House Officer (SHO) for one year before they can become fully registered. Six months of this time will be spent on medical wards and six months on surgical wards
- For new patients, HO's will have results, x-rays and notes ready to discuss with the Consultant as well as the patient's previous medical background, present therapy and how they are progressing
- During ward rounds, HO's update Consultants on patients' recent developments and what the future plans of action are

Senior House Officers (SHO's)

- Fully registered doctors who have completed one year pre-registration (ie their names appear on the medical registry)
- Can work independently and don't have to be supervised to make management decisions, but are still accountable to Consultants
- Train pre-registration doctors and help with the HO's daily tasks
- Take O/P clinics

Registrars

- Help and advise SHO's. Take O/P clinics

Consultants

- Highest senior level. Specialise in a specific area. Take O/P clinics. Train Registrars, SHO's, HO's and manage specific wards (where applicable)

The Medical Team - Nurses

- There are usually three nursing shifts: early (7.30 am - 3.30 pm), late (1.15 pm - 9.00 pm) and night (8.45 pm - 8.00 am). These will vary from hospital to hospital
- Commonly, patient care is split by coded nursing teams for each ward, eg by using colour codes. This is usually outlined on a ward board as well (eg by using colour pens or sections)
- Always try and speak to the specific nurse dealing with your patient (if unsure ask, usually nurses will point you in the right direction)
- Clinical nurse specialists are nurses with special expertise. These include diabetes, respiratory, stoma care, breast care, tissue viability, infection control, symptom control, pain, palliative care and paediatric nurse specialists
- Health Care Assistants (HCA's) help nursing staff with their daily tasks

Professions allied to medicine (PAMs)

- Commonly you will see Physiotherapists, Speech and Language Therapists, Occupational Therapists, Podiatrists and Pharmacists who are also involved with patient care
- Radiographers may also come up to the wards with their radiography equipment to take x-rays of immobile patients

General Ward Information

- Typically, near the nurse's desk on the wards, a board on the wall will list all the patients and bed numbers for the ward
- Meal times: these include breakfast at around 8.00 am, lunch 12.00 noon and evening meal 6.00 pm
- Drug times are usually at 6.00 am, 9.00 am 2.00 pm and 10.00 pm
- Generally speaking, anytime during meal times is not a good time to see a patient, unless you wish to observe meal distribution at ward level or a patient's dietary intake. Apart from interrupting a patient eating, nurses are too busy distributing food and drugs. Try mid morning or mid afternoon instead
- Sometimes it is necessary to follow a ward round when you are particularly concerned about a patient you may be seeing. During clinical placement you will probably be involved with some of these

Medical Notes - An overview

- A patient will enter hospital either by Accident and Emergency (ie unexpected or acute urgency admission) or by their GP/Consultant (ie a planned admission either for further tests and/or an operation)
- For a planned admission the GP will write a letter to the Consultant explaining the patient's problem asking him/her for their medical/surgical opinion. This letter is usually kept

at the back of the patient's medical notes and is useful to look at for a summary of the patient's medical background and current condition

- If the patient was referred via A&E this will usually be documented on an A4 carbon copied sheet at the front of the notes, documenting the patient's details and provisional diagnosis

- This means patients have two separate medical notes, one held at the GP's practice and one in hospital

- Each patient's medical notes are divided into logical sections. Firstly current medical documentation, previous medical documentations (sectioned according to Consultant or medical speciality), correspondences and investigations such as cytology, biochemistry, radiology etc. Some hospitals also hold investigation results on computer

  Inpatients medical notes will be stored in a trolley at ward level, which may be in use during ward rounds

NB The above system will vary, according to hospitals

Medical Notes - Content outline

When a patient is newly admitted, a full medical examination will be done by the appropriate physician. This consists of the following:

- Date admitted
- Source of admittance (ie A&E, GP or Consultant)
- Present condition (PC)
- Past medical condition (PMC) or past medical history (PMH), usually dated list of previous medical conditions
- Social history (SH), ie genetic, inherited factors, what parents died of (if applicable), type of housing/social support and present employment
- Drug history (DH) ie drugs required previously/recent medical conditions such as diabetes, asthma

- Complaining of (CO), present symptoms
- General examination (chest, respiratory function, muscular/ bone movement)
- Plan of action, (tests ordered, referral to PAMs etc)

From here on, plans of action decided by the doctors will be dated and briefly written in the patient's medical notes during ward rounds.

Throughout the medical notes, doctors will use abbreviations like the above, so it is helpful to familiarise yourself with them. (refer to page 110)

Dietetic documentation in the medical notes

- Every dietitian has their own way of writing dietetic information in the medical notes. By the end of placement you will also have developed your own technique. There are no right or wrong ways, but bear in mind the following guidelines:

1. Always date and sign your entry
2. Always begin with 'thank you for referral .....' for newly referred patients. This is considered good manners or of hospital etiquette
3. Never write in pencil or red ink (you are legally required to use black ink)
4. Write legibly and clearly
5. Use correct spelling
6. Avoid dietetic abbreviations (they may be misinterpreted by medical staff)
7. Be specific and to the point
8. Never use correction fluid

- Here are two examples of recording a new dietetic referral for a 79 year old female I/P with malnutrition and Chronic Obstructive Airways Disease (COAD)

Example 1

Date seen by Student Dietitian

Thank you for referral of this 79 year malnourished woman with COAD.

Assessment		**Requirements**
Height:	1.5 M	1700kcal/d
Weight:	55 kg	50 - 60g Protein/d
BMI:	18	

Patient reports weight loss of 3kg over the past month. Due to her tiredness and drowsiness she is currently managing <600kcals and 30g Protein daily.

Recommendations

1. 2 - 3 Ensure Plus/d (providing total 900kcal, 35g protein)

2. High energy and protein foods ordered

3. Small frequent meals/snacks

To review food intake and weight.

Signature
(Student Dietitian)

Example 2 - SOAP Guidelines

Date seen by Student Dietitian

Subjective

Thank you for referring this 79 year old woman with malnutrition and COAD. Due to her tiredness and drowsiness she is currently managing <600kcal/d and 30g protein daily.

Objective

Height: 1.5M   Weight: 55kg   BMI: 18

Current nutritional intake: energy <600kcal/d protein:~30g/d

Assessment

Insufficient dietary intake to meet nutritional requirements. BMI of 18 suggests that this patient is moderately protein and energy depleted.

Plan

To encourage two to three Ensure Plus/d, providing a total of 900kcal and 35g Protein. Suitable high energy/protein meals have also been ordered. I feel this patient would benefit from having small frequent meals/snacks rather than three large meals a day. I have encouraged this and will continue to monitor the patient's progress, regularly.

Signature
(Student Dietitian)

For reviews or follow ups, briefly outline any progress or changes in dietary prescription and date/sign entry.

Nursing Records

- Nurses have a separate written system for documenting patients' details similar to the medical notes. However, nurses do not write in the medical notes

- For each patient, nurses fill out forms which detail their particulars

- Each patient will have a 'care plan' which outlines how the patient is being looked after/any changes

- It is useful to write in the nursing records a brief outline of what you have done so that during 'change overs' all nurses have a written record to refer to

- Nursing details of all patients are combined in one or two folders or separate folders for each patient

Dietetic records

- Dietetic cards vary in style and size but fundamentally record similar patient's details

- Dietetic cards may be colour coded according to dietetic speciality eg diabetics, renal, paediatrics etc

- Blank lines on the back of the card, or on continuation cards allow you to date and document relevant details which may include: blood biochemistry, weight, height, BMI, fluid balance, bowel movement, patients well being/social support, increased/decreased mobility, tests/ investigations, diet history and dietary advice

- Every time you see a patient these details, where appropriate, should be reviewed to assess any changes which may affect dietary intake

- If a patient is to be discharged from hospital, document going home date and state whether an O/P or any other follow up appointment is to be made for them

- Dietitians may also use dietetic records to aid in completing 'statistic records'. Statistic records are increasingly being used in hospitals to retain specific data, eg monthly totals of patients seen by individual Departments

Further reading

Aronson V (1986)
Dietetic Technician: Effective Nutrition Counselling, Avi Pub Co

Billon W E (1991)
Clinical Nutrition Case Studies, West Pub Co, USA

British Dietetic Association (BDA) (1979)
Guidelines for taking diet histories, working party for the BDA

BDA (1992)
Towards the 21st Century. Education and training strategy. Birmingham, UK: BDA

BDA (1991)
Student training pack: Council for professions supplementary to medicine (Dietitians Board)

Gable J (1997)
Counselling skills for Dietitians, Blackwell Science

Hollis B B and Calabrese R J (1991)
Communication and education skills: The dietitians guide, 2nd Edition, Len and Febiger

Judd P A (1996)
Educating the dietitians of the future, Journal of Human Nutrition and Dietetics, **9** pp 333 - 338

Kirby D F, Dudrick, Stanley J (1994)
Practical Handbook of Nutrition in Clinical Practice, CRC P

Labadarios D, Haffejee A (1997)
Handbook of Clinical Nutrition, Oxf VP (S Africa)

Moore MC (1996)
Pocket Guide to Nutrition: Health and Clinical Care, Mosby

Rogers A and Judd P A (1996)
Current and future training of dietitians in th UK - results of the pre-registration working group survey, Journal of Human Nutrition and Dietetics **9** (poster summary, p1)

Wahlqvist, Vobecky M, Jikta S (1986)
Patient problems in Clinical Nutrition: A Manual. J Libbey

Weinsier, Roland L, Butterworth C E, Heimburger D C (1996)
Handbook of Clinical Nutrition: Clinicians Manual of Diagnosis and Management, Mosby

Section 2

Anthropometry

Anthropometry - An overview

- Anthropometry is the technique of expressing qualitatively the form of the body
- Height (metres) and weight (kg) are the most commonly used parameters, since when combined they establish:

  Body Mass Index (BMI)

  Energy requirements (eg to use Schofield Equation requires a patient's weight)

  Gain/loss in weight

  Weight gain/loss necessary to meet ideal body weight

- Body weight is the sum of water, fat, protein, minerals and glycogen
- As a guide, for a 74kg male, approximate body compartments will weigh: water 42kg, fat 15kg, protein 12.8g, minerals and glycogen 4.2g
- Body weight, initially, is a useful measurement of nutritional status: since short term the skeleton is little affected by changes in nutritional status. Therefore, initial weight loss will reflect changes in body fat/protein/water composition
- Conditions such as dehydration, ascites, oedema and large surgical amputations will, however, distort weight readings
- Weighing equipment includes the 'two balance arm principle', electronic/manual scales and chair or hoist scales
- Some times it is impractical to weigh an I/P so try to estimate an approximate weight (check to see whether patient/carer/ nurse may already know this)
- Frequently, height also has to be estimated (as a guide the length of a hospital bed equals approximately 2m/6ft 7"). Alternatively (as an approximate guide) the span of the arms (middle finger to middle finger) can give a rough estimate of height, ie demispan x 2
- Always convert feet into metres and stones into kilograms
- Dietitians may most frequently use height and weight measurements. However, there are other parameters such as body fat and lean body tissue which can be measured to reflect the nutritional status and body composition of a patient (refer fig 2.1)

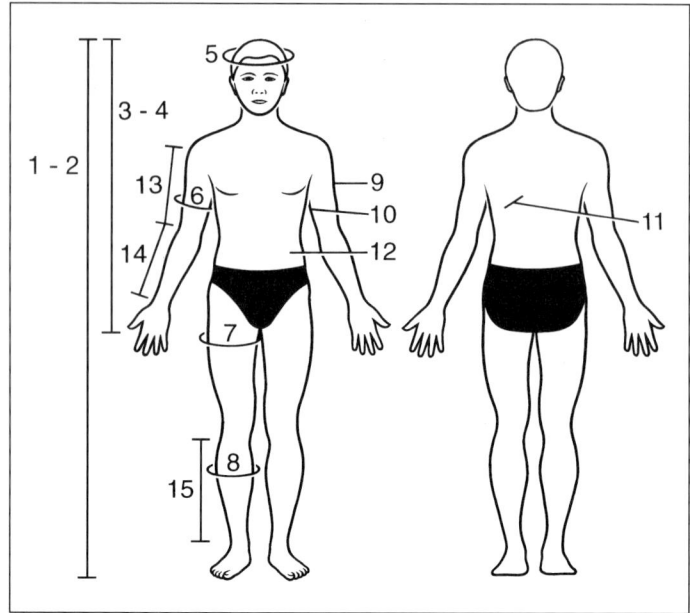

Figure 2.1 - Anthropometric Sites

Key

1 - 2	stature - recumbent length
3 - 4	sitting height (crown-rump length)
5	head circumference
6	upper-arm circumferences
7	upper-thigh circumference
8	maximum calf muscle
9	triceps skinfold
10	biceps skinfold
11	subscapular skinfold
12	supra-iliac skinfold
13	upper arm length
14	forearm length
15	tibial length

Table 2.1 - Height conversion table

ft	in	m	ft	in	m
1	0	0.31	5	5	1.65
2	0	0.61	5	6	1.68
3	0	0.91	5	7	1.70
4	0	1.22	5	8	1.73
4	1	1.25	5	9	1.75
4	2	1.27	5	10	1.78
4	3	1.30	5	11	1.80
4	4	1.32	6	0	1.83
4	5	1.35	6	1	1.85
4	6	1.37	6	2	1.88
4	7	1.40	6	3	1.90
4	8	1.42	6	4	1.93
4	9	1.45	6	5	1.96
4	10	1.47	6	6	1.98
4	11	1.50	6	7	2.01
5	0	1.52	6	8	2.03
5	1	1.55	6	9	2.06
5	2	1.58	6	10	2.08
5	3	1.60	6	11	2.11
5	4	1.63	7	0	2.13

2

Source: British Standards Institute, reproduced with permission. Copies of the chart available by post from BSI Sales, Linford Wood, Milton Keynes, UK.

Height Metric Conversions

1ft	=	30.48 cm	1m	=	39.37 in
1in	=	2.54 cm	1cm	=	0.394 in

Table 2.2 - Weight conversion table - stones and pounds to kilograms

Pounds

Stones	0	1	2	3	4	5	6	7	8	9	10	11	12	13
0		0.45	0.91	1.36	1.81	2.27	2.72	3.18	3.63	4.08	4.54	4.98	5.44	5.89
1	6.35	6.80	7.26	7.71	8.16	8.62	9.07	9.53	9.98	10.43	10.89	11.33	11.79	12.24
2	12.70	13.15	13.61	14.06	14.51	14.97	15.42	15.88	16.33	16.78	17.24	17.68	18.12	18.59
3	19.05	19.50	19.96	20.41	20.86	21.32	21.77	22.23	22.68	23.13	23.59	24.03	24.49	24.94
4	25.40	25.85	26.31	26.76	27.21	27.67	28.12	28.58	29.03	29.48	29.94	30.38	30.84	31.29
5	31.75	32.20	32.66	33.11	33.56	34.02	34.47	34.93	35.38	35.83	36.29	36.73	37.19	37.64
6	38.10	38.55	39.01	39.46	39.91	40.37	40.82	41.28	41.73	42.18	42.64	43.08	43.54	43.99
7	44.45	44.90	45.36	45.81	46.26	46.72	47.17	47.63	48.08	48.53	48.99	49.43	49.89	50.34
8	50.80	51.25	51.71	52.16	52.61	53.07	53.52	53.98	54.43	54.88	55.34	55.78	56.24	56.69
9	57.15	57.60	58.06	58.51	58.96	59.42	59.87	60.33	60.78	61.23	61.69	62.13	62.59	63.04
10	63.50	63.95	64.41	64.86	65.31	65.77	66.22	66.68	67.13	67.58	68.04	68.48	68.94	69.39
11	69.85	70.30	70.76	71.21	71.66	72.12	72.57	73.03	73.48	73.93	74.39	74.83	75.39	75.74
12	76.20	76.65	77.11	77.56	78.01	78.47	78.92	79.38	79.83	80.28	80.74	81.18	81.64	82.09
13	82.55	83.00	83.46	83.91	84.36	84.82	85.27	85.73	86.18	86.63	86.99	87.53	87.99	88.44
14	88.90	89.35	89.81	90.26	90.71	91.17	91.62	92.08	92.53	92.98	93.44	93.88	94.34	94.79
15	95.25	95.70	96.16	96.61	97.06	97.52	97.97	98.43	98.88	99.33	99.79	100.23	100.69	101.14
16	101.60	102.05	102.51	102.96	103.41	103.87	104.32	104.78	105.23	105.68	106.14	106.58	107.04	107.49
17	107.95	108.40	108.86	109.31	109.76	110.22	110.67	111.13	111.58	112.03	112.49	112.93	113.39	113.84
18	114.30	114.75	115.21	115.66	116.11	116.57	117.02	117.48	117.93	118.38	118.84	119.28	119.74	120.19

Source : British Standards Institute, reproduced with permission.

Weight conversion factors   1 stone = 14lbs   = 6.3kg   1kg = 2.2lb

To convert weights > 120kg (18 stone, 13 lbs): kilograms→stones and lbs = weight (kg) ÷ 6.3
Stones and lbs→kilograms = weight (stones and lbs) x 6.3

Body Mass Index (BMI)

- Quetelet index or body mass index:

$$\text{BMI} = \frac{\text{Weight (kg)}}{\text{Height (m}^2)}$$

- BMI expresses grades of obesity in adults (ref table 2.3)

- Round values off to the nearest whole number

Table 2.3 - Grades of obesity

Grade	BMI Range	Comments
	< 12	Death
	< 18	Very underweight
	< 18 - 20	Underweight
	20 - 25	Desirable weight range
1	30 - 35	Overweight
2	35 - 40	Very overweight
3	> 40	Severely overweight

Source: Garrow and Webster (1985)

Calculating percentage of weight loss

$$\frac{\text{usual weight - current weight}}{\text{usual weight}} \times 100$$

Table 2.4 - Desirable weight/height in adults (men)

Average weight in kilograms and pounds (indoor clothing)

Height (in shoes)			Age (years)												
			17 - 19 yrs		20 - 24 yrs		25 - 29 yrs		30 - 39 yrs		40 - 49 yrs		50 - 59 yrs		60 - 69 yrs	
cm	ft	in	kg	lb	kg	lb	kg	lb	kg	lb	kg	lb	kg	lb	kg	lb
157.5	5	2	54	119	58.1	128	60.8	134	62.1	137	63.5	140	64.4	142	63	139
160	5	3	55.8	123	59.9	132	62.6	138	64	141	65.3	144	65.8	145	64.4	142
162.6	5	4	57.6	127	61.7	136	64	141	65.8	145	67.1	148	67.6	149	66.2	146
165.1	5	5	59.4	131	63	139	65.3	144	67.6	149	68.9	152	69.4	153	68	150
167.6	5	6	61.2	135	64.4	142	67.1	148	69.4	153	70.8	156	71.2	157	69.9	154
170.2	5	7	63	139	65.8	145	68.5	151	71.2	157	73	161	73.5	162	72.1	159
172.7	5	8	64.9	143	67.6	149	70.3	155	73	161	74.8	165	75.3	166	73.9	163
175.3	5	9	66.7	147	69.4	153	72.1	159	74.8	165	76.7	169	77.1	170	76.2	168
177.8	5	10	68.5	151	71.2	157	73.9	163	77.1	170	78.9	174	79.4	175	78.5	173
180.3	5	11	70.3	155	73	161	75.8	167	78.9	174	80.8	178	81.6	180	80.8	178
182.9	6	0	72.6	160	75.3	166	78	172	81.2	179	83	183	83.9	185	83	183
185.4	6	1	74.4	164	77.1	170	80.3	177	83	183	84.8	187	85.7	189	85.3	188
188	6	2	76.2	168	78.9	174	82.6	182	85.3	188	87.1	192	88	194	87.5	193
190.5	6	3	78	172	80.8	178	84.4	186	87.5	193	89.4	197	90.3	199	89.8	198
193	6	4	79.8	176	82.1	181	86.2	190	90.3	199	92.1	203	93	205	92.5	204

Source: Entwistle (1992)

Table 2.5 - Desirable weight/height in adults (women)

Average weight in kilograms and pounds (indoor clothing)

Height (in shoes)			Age (years)														
			17 - 19 yrs		20 - 24 yrs		25 - 29 yrs		30 - 39 yrs		40 - 49 yrs		50 - 59 yrs		60 - 69 yrs	
cm	ft	in	kg	lb	kg	lb	kg	lb	kg	lb	kg	lb	kg	lb	kg	lb
147.3	4	10	44.9	99	46.3	102	48.5	107	52.2	115	55.3	122	56.7	125	57.6	127
149.9	4	11	46.3	102	47.6	105	49.9	110	53.1	117	56.2	124	57.6	127	58.5	129
152.4	5	0	47.6	105	49	108	51.3	113	54.4	120	57.6	127	59	130	59.4	131
154.9	5	1	49.4	109	50.8	112	52.6	116	55.8	123	59	130	60.3	133	60.8	134
157.5	5	2	51.3	113	52.2	115	54	119	57.2	126	60.3	133	61.7	136	62.1	137
160	5	3	52.6	116	53.5	118	55.3	122	58.5	129	61.7	136	63.5	140	64	141
162.6	5	4	54.4	120	54.9	121	56.7	125	59.9	132	63.5	140	65.3	144	65.8	145
165.1	5	5	56.2	124	56.7	125	58.5	129	61.2	135	64.9	143	67.1	148	67.6	149
167.6	5	6	57.6	127	58.5	129	60.3	133	63	139	66.7	147	68.9	152	69.4	153
170.2	5	7	59	130	59.9	132	61.7	136	64.4	142	68.5	151	70.8	156	71.2	157
172.7	5	8	60.8	134	61.7	136	63.5	140	66.2	146	70.3	155	72.6	160	73	161
175.3	5	9	62.6	138	63.5	140	65.3	144	68	150	72.1	159	74.4	164	74.8	165
177.8	5	10	64.4	142	65.3	144	67.1	148	69.9	154	74.4	164	76.7	169	-	-
180.3	5	11	66.7	147	67.6	149	69.4	153	72.1	159	76.7	169	78.9	174	-	-
182.9	6	0	68.9	152	69.9	154	71.7	158	74.4	164	78.9	174	81.6	180	-	-

Source: Entwistle (1992)

2

Table 2.6 - Desirable weight/height in children

Average weight in kilograms and pounds

Boys				Age	Girls			
Height		Weight			Height		Weight	
cm	in	kg	lb	(yrs)	cm	in	kg	lb
75.2	29.6	10.1	22.2	1	74.2	29.2	9.8	21.5
87.5	34.4	12.6	27.7	2	86.6	34.1	12.3	27.1
96.2	37.9	14.6	32.2	3	95.7	37.7	14.4	31.8
103.4	40.7	16.5	36.4	4	103.2	40.6	16.4	36.2
111.3	43.8	19.4	42.8	5	109.7	43.2	18.8	41.4
117.5	46.3	21.9	48.3	6	115.9	45.6	21.1	46.5
124.1	48.9	24.5	54.1	7	122.3	48.1	23.7	52.2
130.0	51.2	27.3	60.1	8	128.0	50.4	26.3	58.1
135.5	53.3	29.9	66.0	9	132.9	52.3	28.9	63.8
140.3	55.2	32.6	71.9	10	138.6	54.6	31.9	70.3
144.2	56.8	35.2	77.6	11	144.7	57.0	35.7	78.8
149.6	58.9	38.3	84.4	12	151.9	59.8	39.7	87.6
155.0	61.0	42.2	93.0	13	157.1	61.9	44.9	99.1
162.7	64.1	48.8	107.6	14	159.6	62.8	49.2	108.4
167.8	66.1	54.5	120.1	15	161.1	63.4	51.5	113.4
171.6	67.6	58.8	129.7	16	162.2	63.9	53.1	117.0

Source: Entwistle (1992)

NB Male and female paediatric centile height and weight charts are also available

Average weight gain in pregnancy

First week - 12 weeks   =   1kg weight gain per week

12 weeks >   =   0.3 - 0.4kg weight gain per week

Total 10-12kg weight gain throughout pregnancy

NB Fluid retention, when present, may distort weight measurments

Table 2.7 - Average weight gain in infancy

Average weight in kiograms, pounds and ounces

Age (weeks)	kg	lbs	ozs	Age (weeks)	kg	lbs	ozs
Birth	3.48	7	11	28	8.14	17	15
4	4.17	9	3	32	8.54	18	13
8	5.08	11	3	36	8.90	19	10
12	5.87	12	15	40	9.22	20	5
16	6.58	14	8	44	9.65	21	4
20	7.14	15	12	48	9.97	22	0
24	7.65	16	14	52	10.21	22	9

Source: Entwistle (1992)

References and Further Reading

Bassey E J (1996)
Anthropometric Tips, International Journal of Obesity and Related Metabolic Disorders 20 (4) pp376

Entwistle I R (1992)
Exacta Medica: Reference Tables and Data For The Medical and Nursing Professions, Churchill Livingstone

Garrow J S; Webster J (1985)
Quetelet's index (w/h^2) as a measure of fatness, International Journal Obesity 9 pp147-53

Gibson R S (1993)
Nutritional Assessment: A Laboratory Manual, Oxford University Press

Gibson R S (1990)
Principles of Nutritional Assessment, Oxford University Press

Gorstein J; Sullivan K; Yipr, De Onis M; Trowbridge E F; Fanjans P; Clugston G (1994)
Issues in the assessment of nutritional status using anthropometry, Bulletin of The World Health Organization 72 (2) pp 273-83

Harrison J E; McNeill K G (1994)
Nutritional assessment review, Blood Purification 12 (1) pp 68-72

Jebbs S A; Elia (1993)
Techniques for the measurement of body composition: a pratical guide, International Journal of Obesity And Related Metabolic Disorders 17 (11) pp 611-21

Jurgens, Hans W (1990)
International data on Anthropometry, ILO Occupational Safety and Health 5

Lohman T G, Roche A E, Martorell R (1988)
Anthropometric Standardization Manual. Human Kinetics Books, Champagne, Illinois

Tanner J M (1966)
Standards from birth to maturity for height, weight, height velocity and weight velocity in British children, Archives of Disease in Childhood 41 pp 454-471, 613-635

Ulijaszek S J, Taylor, Mascie C G N (1994)
Anthropometry: The individual and the population, Camp, UP, Cambridge Studies in Biological Anthropology

World Health Organisation (WHO) (1996)
Physical Status: Use and interpretation of Anthropometry, WHO Technical Report 5, No. 854

Section 3

Nutritional Requirements

Calculating energy requirements for adults (using Schofield Equation)

NB The following method gives a detailed calculation for estimating a patient's energy requirement. This is most commonly used for adult patients receiving artificial nutritional support. For a quick guide refer to Table 3.4

1. Determine patient's Basal Metabolic Rate (BMR) either by approximate guide (Table 3.1) or Schofield equation (Table 3.2)

3

Table 3.1 - Approximate guide to estimating BMR

KG	KCAL/Day	KG	KCAL/Day
35	950	70	1550
40	1000	75	1650
45	1050	80	1700
50	1200	85	1800
55	1300	90	1850
60	1400	95	1950
65	1450	100	2000

Source: Taylor and Goodinson-McLaren (1992)

Table 3.2 - Schofield equation

Age (yrs)	Male	Female
15 - 18	BMR=17.6 x weight (kg) + 656	BMR=13.3 x weight (kg) + 690
18 - 30	BMR=15.0 x weight (kg) + 690	BMR=14.8 x weight (kg) + 485
30 - 60	BMR=11.4 x weight (kg) + 870	BMR=8.1 x weight (kg) + 842
> 60	BMR=11.7 x weight (kg) + 585	BMR=9.0 x weight (kg) + 656

Source: Schofield (1985)

2. To BMR add:

   A) Stress Factor (refer to Fig 3.1)

   B) Activity and diet-induced thermogenesis

Bedbound immobile	-	+10%
Bedbound mobile/sitting	-	+15 - 20%
Mobile on ward	-	+25%

   C) Add or subtract up to 400 - 1000kcal/d if weight gain/ loss is required (weight loss not applicable for severely ill patients)

Source: Adapted from Todorvic V and Micklewright A (1997).

Table 3.3 - Estimating energy requirements (EER) for adults (using Harris-Benedict Equation)

Men	Women
EER (kcal = 66.5 + 13.75W + 5.00H - 6.77A	EER (kcal) = 655.1 + 9.56W + 1.85H - 4.67A
EER (kJ) = 278 + 57.5W + 20.93H - 28.35A	EER (kJ) = 2741 + 40.0W + 7.74H - 19.56A

Source: Harris and Benedict (1991)

W = weight (kg)   H = height (cm)   A = age (years)

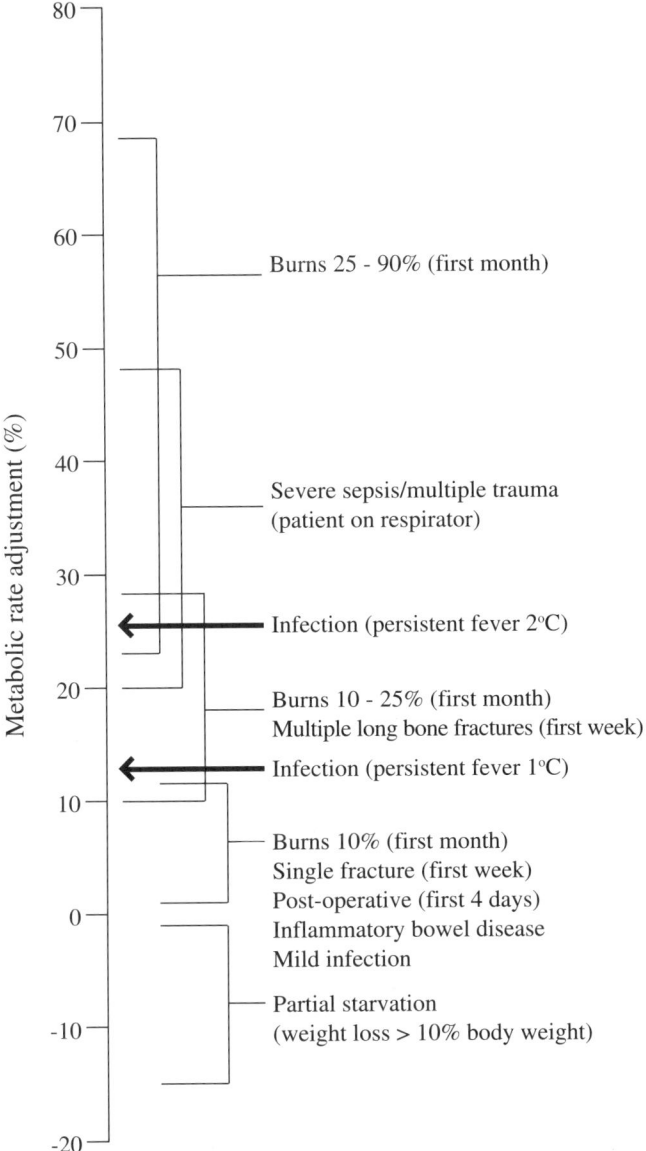

Fig 3.1 Elia Normagram
Source: Elia (1990). Reproduced with permission

Table 3.4 - PENG guidelines for general [1]adult nutritional requirements

Metabolic state	Energy kcal/kg (KJ)	Protein g/kg	Nitrogen g/kg	[2]Fluid ml/kg	Sodium mmol/kg	Potassium mmol/g Nitrogen	Phosphate mmol/day
Normal up to 25%	30	1.0 (125)	0.16	30 - 35	1.0 (min 50 total per day)	5.0	20
Intermediate 25 - 55%	35-40 (150 - 170)	1.3 - 1.9	0.2 - 0.3	30 - 35	1.0	5.0	20-30
Hypermetabolic 45 - 100%	40-60 (170 - 150)	2-3	0.3 - 0.5	30 - 35	1.0	7.0	Max 50

Source: Todorovic V and Micklewright A (1989). Reproduced with kind permission.

[1] per kg Actual Body Weight

[2] Add 2 - 2.5 ml/kg/day for each °C rise in body temperature above 37°C

Additional notes - Table 3.4

- For patients with a BMI > 30 use 75% of estimated protein requirements
- Always make provision for renal losses and non-renal losses eg diarrhoea and fistulas on an individual basis

For each 1^0C rise in temperature in addition to above add:

- 0.6g Nitrogen (with sweating)
- 30 mmol Na
- 10% energy requirments
- 500 - 750 ml fluid

Potassium

- 5 mmol per g/Nitrogen = minimum requirement for maximum protein utilisation
- Serum K levels depleted (below 3.5 mmol/l) additional 2 mmol g/N
- refeeding severely malnourished patients add 2 mmol g/N

UK Dietary Reference Values

- Recommended daily intakes (RDI) and recommended daily amounts (RDA) are the old values for defining the adequacy of diets for the majority of the UK population
- The current system uses dietary reference values (DRV's) which cover the following categories (DOH, 1991):
  1. Estimated average requirements (EAR's) - used for main energy yielding nutrients such as fats, sugars, starches, Non-Starch Polysaccharides as well as estimating energy requirements. About half of the population usually need more than the EAR, and half less
  2. Reference nutrient intakes (RNI), equivalent to the old RDA or RDI values, are adequate for 97% of the UK population. The risk of deficiency in this group is very small
  3. Lower Reference Nutrient Intake (LNRI) for protein, vitamins and minerals. An amount of the nutrient that is sufficient for only a few people in a group who have lower needs

4. Safe intake. Term used to indicate intake or range of intakes of a nutrient for which there is not enough information to estimate RNI, EAR or LRNI. An amount that is enough for almost everyone but not so large as to cause undesirable effects

Table 3.5 - Estimated Average Requirements for Energy

EARs in MJ/d (kcal/d)

Age	Males	Females
0 - 3 months	2.28 (545)	2.16 (515)
4 - 6 months	2.89 (690)	2.69 (645)
7 - 9 months	3.44 (825)	3.20 (765)
10 - 12 months	3.85 (920)	3.61 (865)
1 - 3 years	5.15 (1,230)	4.86 (1,165)
4 - 6 years	7.16 (1,715)	6.46 (1,545)
7 - 10 years	8.24 (1,970)	7.28 (1,740)
11 - 14 years	9.27 (2,220)	7.92 (1,845)
15 - 18 years	11.51 (2,775)	8.83 (2,110)
19 - 50 years	10.60 (2,550)	8.10 (1,940)
51 - 59 years	10.60 (2,550)	8.00 (1,900)
60 - 64 years	9.93 (2,380)	7.99 (1,900)
65 - 74 years	9.71 (2,330)	7.96 (1,900)
75+ years	8.77 (2,100)	7.61 (1,810)
Pregnancy		+0.80*(200)
Lactation		
1 month		+1.90 (450)
2 months		+2.20 (530)
3 months		+2.40 (570)
4 - 6 months (Group 1)		+2.00 (480)
4 - 6 months (Group 2)		+2.40 (570)
>6 months (Group 1)		+1.00 (240)
>6 months (Group 2)		+2.30 (550)

Source: DOH (1991) Crown copyright is reproduced with the permission of the Controller of HMSO.

*last trimester only

34

Table 3.6 - Reference Nutrient Intakes for Protein

Age	Reference Nutrient Intake[a] (g/d)
0 - 3 months	12.5[b]
4 - 6 months	12.7
7 - 9 months	13.7
10 - 12 months	14.9
1 - 3 years	14.5
4 - 6 years	19.7
7 - 10 years	28.3
Males	
11 - 14 years	42.1
15 - 18 years	55.2
19 - 50 years	55.5
50+ years	53.3
Females	
11 - 14 years	41.2
15 - 18 years	45.0
19 - 50 years	45.0
50+ years	46.5
Pregnancy[c]	+ 6
Lactation[c]	
0 - 4 months	+ 11
4+ months	+ 8

3

Source: DOH (1991) Crown copyright is reproduced with the permission of the Controller of HMSO.

a These figures, based on egg and milk protein, assume complete digestibility

b No values for infants 0 - 3 months are given by WHO. The RNI is calculated from the recommendations of COMA

c To be added to adult requirement through all stages of pregnancy and lactation

Table 3.7 - Adult Diatary Reference Values for fat and carbohydrate (as a percentage of daily total energy intake/percentage of food energy)

Nutrient	Individual minimum		Population average	Individual maximum
Saturated fatty acids			10 (11)	
Cis-polyunsaturated fatty acids	n - 3 n - 6	0.2 1.0	6 (6.5)	10
Cis-monounsaturated fatty acids			12 (13)	
Trans fatty acids			2 (2)	
Total fatty acids			30 (32.5)	
Total fat			**33 (35)**	
Non-milk extrinsic sugars	0		10 (11)	
Intrinsic and milk sugars and starch			37 (39)	
Total carbohydrate			**47 (50)**	
Non-starch Polysaccharide (g/d)	**12**		**18**	**24**

Source: DOH (1991) Crown copyright is reproduced with the permission of the Controller of HMSO.

Table 3.8 - Adult Reference Nutrient Intakes for vitamins

Age	Thiamin mg/d	Riboflavin mg/d	Niacin (nicotinic acid equivalent mg/d	Vit. B6 mg/d†	Vit. B12 µg/d	Folate µg/d	Vit. C mg/d	Vit. A µg/d	Vit. D µg/d
0 - 3 mths	0.2	0.4	3	0.2	0.3	50	25	350	8.5
4 - 6 mths	0.2	0.4	3	0.2	0.3	50	25	350	8.5
7 - 9 mths	0.2	0.4	4	0.3	0.4	50	25	350	7
10 - 12 mths	0.3	0.4	5	0.4	0.4	50	25	350	7
1 - 3 yrs	0.5	0.6	8	0.7	0.5	70	30	400	7
4 - 6 yrs	0.7	0.8	11	0.9	0.8	100	30	500	-
7 - 10 yrs	0.7	1.0	12	1.0	1.0	150	30	500	-
Males									
11 - 14 yrs	0.9	1.2	15	1.2	1.2	200	35	600	-
15 - 18 yrs	1.1	1.3	18	1.5	1.5	200	40	700	-
19 - 50 yrs	1.0	1.3	17	1.4	1.5	200	40	700	-
50+ yrs	0.9	1.3	16	1.4	1.5	200	40	700	**
Females									
11 - 14 yrs	0.7	1.1	12	1.0	1.2	200	35	600	-
15 - 18 yrs	0.8	1.1	14	1.2	1.5	200	40	600	-
19 - 50 yrs	0.8	1.1	13	1.2	1.5	200	40	600	-
50+ yrs	0.9	1.1	12	1.2	1.5	200	40	600	**
Pregnancy	+0.1***	+0.3	*	*	*	+100	+10	+100	10
Lactation									
0 - 4 mths	+0.2	+0.5	+2	*	+0.5	+60	+30	+350	10
4+ mths	+0.2	+0.5	+2	*	+0.5	+60	+30	+350	10

Source: DOH (1991) Crown copyright is reproduced with the permission of the Controller of HMSO

* no increment ** after age 65 RNI is 10µg/d for men and women ***for last trimester only

† based on protein providing 14.7% of EAR for energy

3

Table 3.9 - Adult Reference Nutrient Intakes for minerals (SI units)

Age	Calcium mmol/d	Phosphorus[1] mmol/d	Magnesium mmol/d	Sodium[2] mmol/d	Potassium[3] mmol/d	Chloride[4] mmol/d	Iron[5] µmmol/d	Zinc µmol/d	Copper µmol/d	Selenium µmol/d	Iodine µmol/d
0 - 3 mths	13.1	13.1	2.2	9	20	9	30	60	5	0.1	0.4
4 - 6 mths	13.1	13.1	2.5	12	22	12	80	60	5	0.2	0.5
7 - 9 mths	13.1	13.1	3.2	14	18	14	140	75	5	0.1	0.5
10 - 12 mths	13.1	13.1	3.3	15	18	15	140	75	5	0.1	0.5
1 - 3 yrs	8.8	8.8	3.5	22	20	22	120	75	6	0.2	0.6
4 - 6 yrs	11.3	11.3	4.8	30	28	30	110	100	9	0.3	0.8
7 - 10 yrs	13.8	13.8	8.0	50	50	50	160	110	11	0.4	0.9
Males											
11 - 14 yrs	25.0	25.0	11.5	70	80	70	200	140	13	0.6	1.0
15 - 18 yrs	25.0	25.0	12.3	70	90	70	200	145	16	0.9	1.0
19 - 50 yrs	17.5	17.5	12.3	70	90	70	160	145	19	0.9	1.0
50+ yrs	17.5	17.5	12.3	70	90	70	160	145	19	0.9	1.0
Females											
11 - 14 yrs	20.0	10.0	11.5	70	80	70	260[5]	140	13	0.6	1.0
15 - 18 yrs	20.0	20.0	12.3	70	90	70	260[5]	110	16	0.8	1.1
19 - 50 yrs	17.5	17.5	10.9	70	90	70	260[5]	110	19	0.8	1.1
50+ yrs	17.5	17.5	10.9	70	90	70	160	110	19	0.8	1.1
Pregnancy	*	*	*	*	*	*	*	*	*	*	*
Lactation											
0 - 4 mths	+14.3	+14.3	+2.1	*	*	*	*	+90	+5	+0.2	*
4+ mths	+14.3	+14.3	+2.1	*	*	*	*	+40	+5	+0.2	*

Source: DOH (1991) Crown copyright reproduced with the permission of the Controller of HMSO

* no increment [1] Phosphorous RNI is set equal to calcium in molar terms [2] 1mmol sodium = 23mg [3] 1mmol potassium = 39mg [4] corresponds to sodium 1mmol = 35.5mg [5] insufficient for women with high menstrual losses where the most practical way of meeting iron requirments is to take an iron supplement

3

Table 3.10 - Adult Reference Nutrient Intakes for minerals (mg/d)

Age	Calcium mg/d	Phosphorus[1] mg/d	Magnesium mg/d	Sodium[2] mg/d	Potassium[3] mg/d	Chloride[4] mg/d	Iron[5] mg/d	Zinc mg/d	Copper mg/d	Selenium µg/d	Iodine µg/d
0 - 3 mths	525	400	55	210	800	320	1.7	4.0	0.2	10	50
4 - 6 mths	525	400	60	280	850	400	4.3	4.0	0.3	13	60
7 - 9 mths	525	400	75	320	700	500	7.8	5.0	0.3	10	60
10 - 12 yrs	525	400	80	350	700	500	7.8	5.0	0.3	10	60
1 - 3 yrs	350	270	85	500	800	800	6.9	5.0	0.4	15	70
4 - 6 yrs	450	350	120	700	1,100	1,100	6.1	6.5	0.6	20	100
7 - 10 yrs	550	450	200	1,200	2,000	1,800	8.7	7.0	0.7	30	110
Males											
11 - 14 yrs	1,000	775	280	1,600	3,100	2,500	11.3	9.0	0.8	45	130
15 - 18 yrs	1,000	775	300	1,600	3,500	2,500	11.3	9.5	1.0	70	140
19 - 50 yrs	700	550	300	1,600	3,500	2,500	8.7	9.5	1.2	75	140
50+ yrs	700	550	300	1,600	3,500	2,500	8.7	9.5	1.2	75	140
Females											
11 - 14 yrs	800	625	280	1,600	3,100	2,500	14.8[5]	9.0	0.8	45	130
15 - 18 yrs	800	625	300	1,600	3,500	2,500	14.8[5]	7.0	1.0	60	140
19 - 50 yrs	700	550	270	1,600	3,500	2,500	14.8[5]	7.0	1.2	60	140
50+ yrs	700	550	270	1,600	3,500	2,500	8.7	7.0	1.2	60	140
Pregnancy	*	*	*	*	*	*	*	*	*	*	*
Lactation											
0 - 4 mths	+550	+440	+50	*	*	*	*	+6.0	+0.3	+15	*
4+ mths	+550	+440	+50	*	*	*	*	+2.5	+0.3	+15	*

Source: DOH (1991) Crown copyright reproduced with the permission of the Controller of HMSO.

* no increment [1] Phosphorous RNI is set equal to calcium in molar terms [2] 1mmol sodium = 23mg [3] 1mmol potassium = 39mg [4] corresponds to sodium 1mmol = 35.5mg [5] insufficient for women with high menstrual losses where the most practical way of meeting iron requirments is to take an iron supplement

Table 3.11 - Adult safe intakes for vitamins and minerals

Nutrient	Safe intake
Vitamins	
Pantothenic acid	
adults	3 - 7 mg/d
infants	1.7 mg/d
Biotin	10 - 200 µg/d
Vitamin E	
men	above 4 mg/d
women	above 3 mg/d
infants	0.4 mg/g polyunsaturated fatty acids
Vitamin K	
adults	1µg/kg/d
infants	10 µg/d
Minerals	
Manganese	
adults	1.4 mg/d (26µmol/d)
infants and children	16 µg/kg/d
Molybdenum	
adults	50 - 400 µg/d
infants, children and adolescents	0.5 - 1.5 µg/kg/d
Chromium	
adults	25 µg (0.5µmol)/d
children and adolescents	0.1 - 1.0 µg (2 - 20µmol) /kg/d
Fluoride (for infants only)	0.05 mg (3µmol)/kg/d

Source: DOH (1991) Crown copyright is reproduced with the permission of the Controller of HMSO.

Table 3.12 - Paediatric selected dietary Reference Nutrient Intakes

Age	Weight kg	Fluid ml/kg	Energy (EAR) kJ/day	kJ/kg/day	kcal/day	kcal/kg/day	Protein g/day	g/kg/day
Males								
0 - 3 mths	4.4	150	2280	480 - 420	545	115 - 100	12.5	2.8
4 - 6	7.2	130	2890	400	690	95	12.7	1.8
7 - 9	9.0	120	3440	400	825	95	13.7	1.5
10 - 12	10.0	110	3850	400	920	95	14.9	1.5
1 - 3 yrs	12.7	95	5150	400	1230	95	14.5	1.1
4 - 6	18.04	85	7160	380	1715	90	19.7	1.1
7 - 10	28.3	75	8240	-	1970	-	28.3	-
11 - 14	43.0	55	9270	-	2220	-	42.1	-
15 - 18	64.5	50	11510	-	2755	-	55.2	-
Females								
0 - 3 mths	4.4	150	2160	480 - 420	515	115 - 100	12.5	2.8
4 - 6	7.2	130	2690	400	645	95	12.7	1.8
7 - 9	9.0	120	3200	400	765	95	13.7	1.5
10 - 12	10.0	110	3610	400	865	95	14.9	1.5
1 - 3 yrs	12.7	95	4860	400	1165	95	14.5	1.1
4 - 6	18.4	85	6460	380	1545	90	19.7	1.1
7 - 10	28.3	75	7280	-	1740	-	28.3	-
11 - 14	43.8	55	7920	-	1845	-	41.2	-
15 - 18	55.5	50	8830	-	2110	-	45.4	-

Source: DOH (1991) Crown copyright is reproduced with the permission of the Controller of HMSO.

3

Table 3.12 - Paediatric selected dietary Reference Nutrient Intakes (cont)

Age	Sodium mmol/day	Sodium mmol/kg/day	Potassium mmol/day	Potassium mmol/kg/day	Vitamin C mg/day	Calcium mmol/day	Iron μmol/day
Males							
0 - 3 mths	9	2.0	20	4.5	25	13.1	30
4 - 6	12	1.7	22	3.1	25	13.1	80
7 - 9	14	1.6	18	2.0	25	13.1	140
10 - 12	15	1.5	18	1.8	25	13.1	140
1 - 3 yrs	22	1.7	20	1.6	30	8.8	120
4 - 6	30	1.6	28	1.5	30	11.3	110
7 - 10	50	-	50	-	30	13.8	160
11 - 14	70	-	80	-	35	25.0	200
15 - 18	70	-	90	-	40	25.0	200
Females							
0 - 3 mths	9	2.0	20	4.5	25	13.1	30
4 - 6	12	1.7	22	3.1	25	13.1	80
7 - 9	14	1.6	18	2.0	25	13.1	140
10 - 12	15	1.5	18	1.8	25	13.1	140
1 - 3 yrs	22	1.7	20	1.6	30	8.8	120
4 - 6	30	1.6	28	1.5	30	11.3	110
7 - 10	50	-	50	-	30	13.8	160
11 - 14	70	-	80	-	35	20.0	260
15 - 18	70	-	90	-	40	20.0	260

3

Source: DOH (1991) Crown copyright is reproduced with the permission of the Controller of HMSO

References and further reading

Chernoff R (1994)
Thirst and fluid requirements, Nutrition Reviews 52 (8) Part 2 pp53-5

Department of Health (1991)
Dietary reference values for food energy and nutrients for the United Kingdom, Soc Subj 41. HMSO, London

Eaton S B; Eaton S B 3rd; Konner M J; Shostak M (1996)
An evolutionary perspective enchances understanding of human nutritional requirements, Journal of Nutrition 126 (6) pp1732-40

Elia M (1990)
Artificial Nutritional Support, Medicine 82 pp3394

Elia M (1992)
Energy Expenditure in the whole body; In energy metabolism: Tissue determinants and cellular corollaries, Raven Press, New York

Fairweather - Tait S J October (1993)
Optimal Nutrient requirements: important concepts, Journal of Human Nutrition and Dietetics, 6 (s), 411 - 419

Harris J A; Benedict F G (1991)
Biometric studies of basal metabolism in man, Carnegic Institute, Washington

Milward D J; Bowtell J L; Pacy P; Renniem M J (1994)
Physical activity, protein metabolism and protein requirements, Proceeding of the Nutrition Society 53 (1) pp223-40

Moe P W (1994)
Future directions for energy requirements and food energy values, Journal of Nutrition 124 (9 Suppl) pp1738S-1742S

Rosenberg I H (1994)
Nutritional requirements for optimal health: what does that mean? Journal of Nutrition 124 (9 Suppl) pp1777S-1779S

3

Schofield W N (1985)
Predicting basal metabolic rate, new standards and reviews of previous work. Hum Nutr Clin Nutr 44 pp1 - 19

Shetty P S; Henry C Y; Black A E; Prentice A M (1996)
Energy requirements of adults: an update on basal metabolic rates and physical activity levels, European Journal of Clinical Nutrition 50 Suppl 1ppS11-23

Taylor S; Goodinson - McLaren (1992)
Nutrition support: A team approach, Wolf Publishing Ltd

Todorovic V and Micklewright A (1989), (1997)
A pocket guide to clinical nutrition 1st Ed and 2nd Ed, Parenteral and Enteral Nutrition Group of The British Dietetic Association

3

Section 4

Enteral Nutrition

Enteral tube feeding

Definition
- Using the gut for the digestion of nutrients via a polyurethene or PVC feeding tube

Indications
- Patients who have a functioning gut but continue to have a poor oral dietary intake (for five days or more) and/or are unable to meet their nutritional requirements from an oral dietary intake alone, eg catabolic patients, head and neck injuries etc

Contra-indications
- Paralytic ileus (absolute contraindication)
- Intestinal obstruction
- Any GI surgery (pre and post op) requiring total bowel rest
- Certain bowel fistulas
- Acute pancreatitis (Naso-Jejunal feeding past the pancreas may be suitable)
- Total blockage of the oesophagus

Examples of common tube fed patients
- Dysphagic patients
- Coma/unconscious patients
- Patients with increased nutritional requirements unable to be met by dietary intake alone (eg burns/trauma/orthopaedic/HIV and surgical patients)
- Early feeding of Low Birth Weight infants
- Chemo/Radiotherapy patients
- Surgical patients (especially head and neck involvement resulting in physical eating problems)
- Depressed patients with prolonged disinterest in food
- Dementia patients

Routes of administration (refer fig 4.1, 4.2 and 4.3)
- Short term - Naso-Gastric, Oro-Gastric, Oesophagastric, Naso-Duodenal, Naso-Jejunal
- Long term - Oesophagastomy, Gastrostomy/PEG, Jejunostomy

4

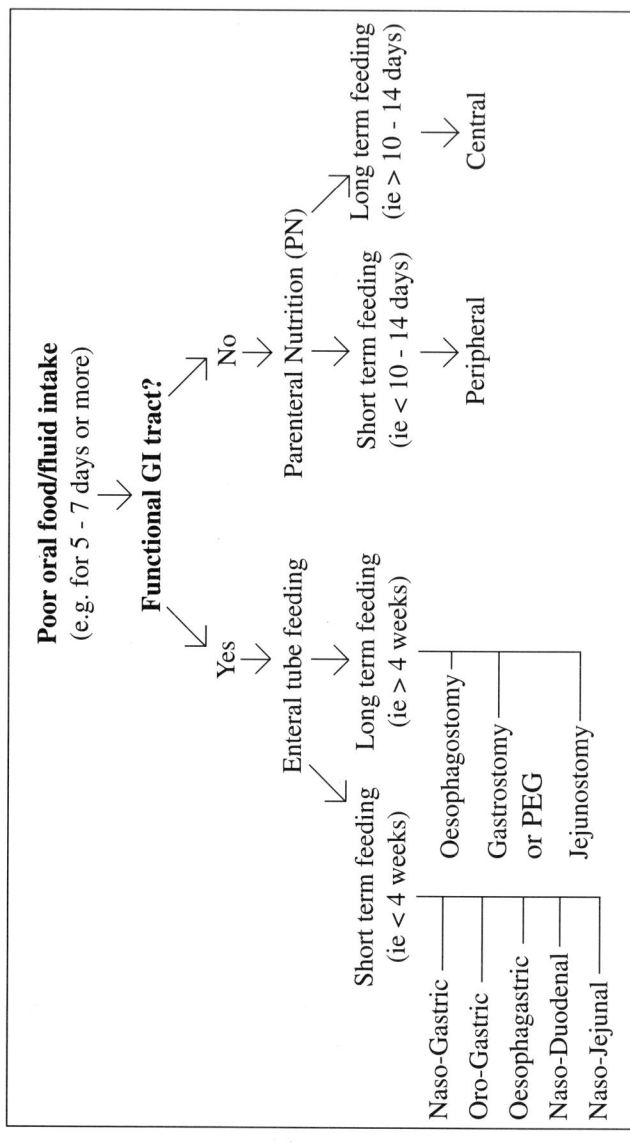

Figure 4.1 - Administration and indications for enteral and parenteral feeding

Administration and indications - enteral tube feeding
Short term - Enteral feeding < 4 weeks
Naso-Gastric (NG)
- For patients who have full use of their stomach

Oro-Gastric (OG)
- Used in head injury patients when extent of damage is unknown and if an NG tube is passed it may go into the inter-cranial space. May also be used for patients with nasal trauma where passing an NG tube would be inappropriate

Oesophagastric
- Used for head and neck patients. Involves placing a fine bore tube through the tracheostomy and an existing tracheo-oesophageal fistulae

Naso-Duodenal (ND)
- For patients who need their stomach to be bypassed

Naso-Jejunal (NJ)
- For patients who need both their stomach and duodenum bypassed, eg patients at risk of aspiration, continual nausea and vomiting and upper GI strictures/obstructions/surgery

Long term - Enteral feeding > 4 weeks
Oesophagostomy (Cervical Pharnyx)
- These tubes are primarily used by surgeons operating on the head and neck. Also known as cervical pharnyx. A fine bore tube is placed surgically through the neck into the oesophagus or pharnyx

Percutaneous endoscopically placed gastrostomy (PEG)
- There are two main types of gastrostomies: a surgical gastrostomy or a PEG. Both are very similar, except a surgical gastrostomy requires a general anaesthetic and laparotomy, whilst a PEG is placed endoscopically under sedation using specially designed kits. PEGs tend to be used now more than surgical gastrostomies and are only contra-indicated if it is impossible to pass an endoscope on the patient.

Jejunostomy
- For patients who require both their stomach and duodenum to be bypassed, refer to the above under NJ

4

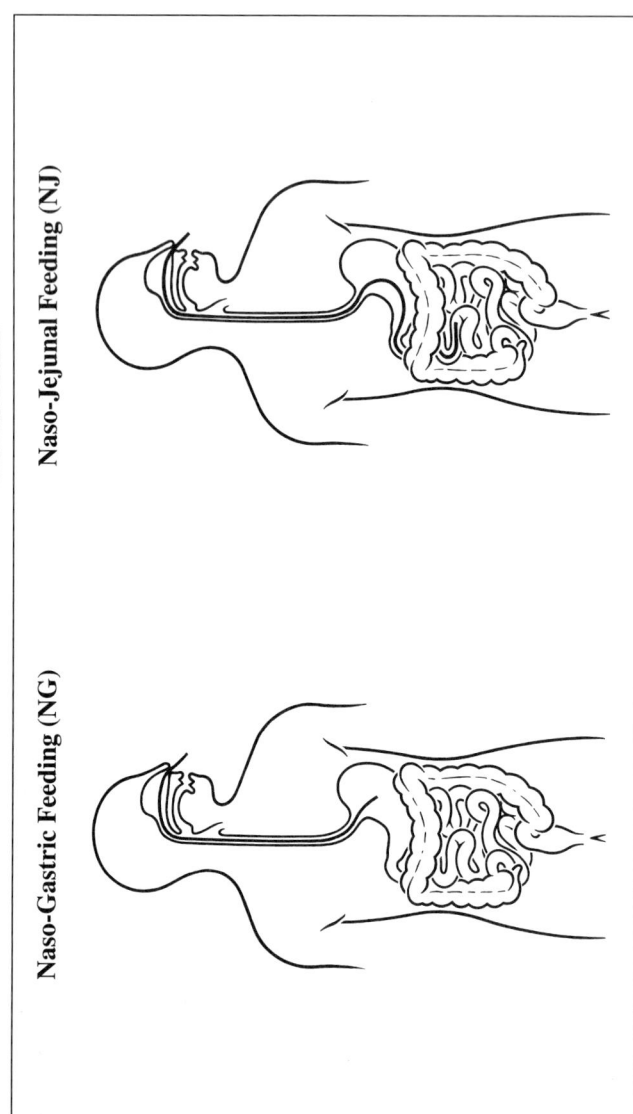

Naso-Gastric Feeding (NG)

Naso-Jejunal Feeding (NJ)

Fig 4.2 Example routes of administration - Short term
Source: Marks and Ponsky (1995)

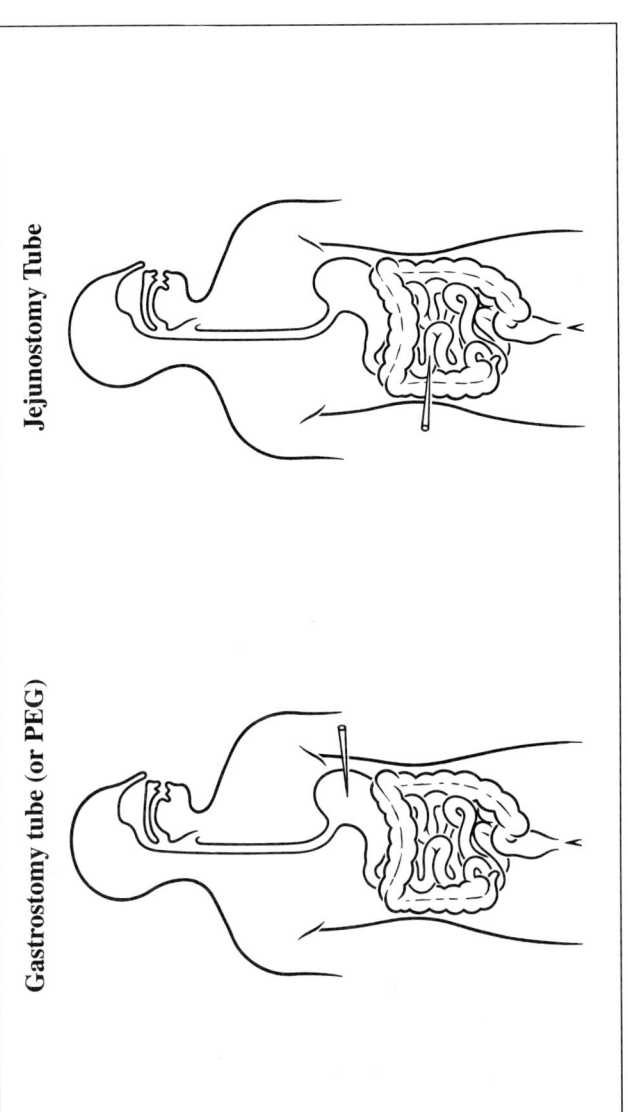

Gastrostomy tube (or PEG)

Jejunostomy Tube

4

Fig 4.3 Example routes of administration - Long term
Source: Marks and Ponsky (1995)

Tube feeding into the stomach

- Avoid tube feeding for more than 18 hours a day (ie allow minimum of 6 hours rest per day). During feeding the pH of the stomach rises. Resting the stomach allows it to return to its normal pH of 2. This helps kill any bacteria present and prevents transmission of gastric organisms to the tracheo bronchial tree thereby reducing the risk of pneumonia

- Complications
  Short term feeding
  - Refer table 4.1

  Long term feeding
  - For gastrostomy/PEG feeding: local wound infection, granulation of tissue, necrotising fascites, intra abdo abcesses. Also refer table 4.1

Tube feeding bypassing the stomach

- Bypassing the stomach means that there is no stomach to act as a 'reservoir' for feed. Therefore try to feed continuously at the lowest rate possible

- Feeds given jejunally may need to be isotonic or semi-elemental (but full strength feeds can be tolerated)

- Diarrhoea occurs frequently in these types of patients so observe the 'plan of action' for this problem in table 4.1

- If diarrhoea continues, send a stool sample to eliminate infection as a cause. If there is no infection, try a fibre containing feed or reducing the feed rate. Consider antidiarrhoeal drugs and check antibiotics and other medications which could cause diarrhoea (refer page 73). The side effects of antibiotics can last up to two weeks post discontinuation

Feeding tubes

1. **Wide bore naso-gastric tubes (Ryles and Levin's tubes)**
   (Manufacturers only guarantee 48 hours to remain in situ)

   - Originally designed for stomach drainage

   - Uncomfortable for patient

   - Can cause oesophageal ulceration

   - Occasionally used in patients with risk of aspiration (eg dysphagic patients) or post operatively where there is concern regarding gastric function

2. **Fine bore naso-gastric tubes**

   - Now most commonly used, since their narrowness and pliability make them more comfortable

   - Range of guages (diameters) available

   - Available in PVC for short term feeding (ie < 10 - 14 days)

   - Available in polyurethane for longer term feeding

   - Guidewire (in some tubes) used to insert tube

Types of infusion feeding

1. **Bolus feeding**

   - 'Infusing' volumes of feed down a feeding tube via a syringe

   - May be used for restless or agitated patients who frequently disconnect giving sets or patients who require additional nutritional supplementation with oral dietary intake.

   - Now rarely used as rapid administration of large volumes of feed is associated with diarrhoea and abdominal discomfort

   - 100 - 300 mls over 10 - 30 mins several times a day

   - No more than 250 - 300 mls feed per infusion

2. **Gravity feeding**
   - Continual drip feeding (by adjusting the roller clamp on the giving set)
   - Drip rate is calculated and adjusted to match the prescribed volume of feed in a set time
   - More time consuming and less accurate than pump feeding

3. **Pump feeding**
   - Feeding pumps are used to control feed rate
   - A variety of pumps are currently available
   - Now most commonly used

Starting pump tube feeding - example of equipment checklist

- Pump and lead (record pump number and record in log book, if applicable)
- NG tube (already placed and checked)
- Giving set (equipment used to attach feed to pump)
- Feed (ready to hangs/bottles, remember flexitainers if need to decant)
- Write Starter regimen (refer Fig 4.4 and 4.5 for examples)

Example of checklist for initiating tube feeding

- Liase nurses/doctors
- Check patients blood biochemistry (eg sodium, potassium, urea, creatinine and albumin)
- Calculate patients Energy, Protein, Sodium, Potassium, Carbohydrate and fluid requirements
- Decide most suitable feeding route
- Decide most suitable feed and volume required

- Calculate pump/drip rate, allowing at least 6 hours rest (if feeding into the stomach)
- Insert tube feeding regimen chart into the patient's bed-end folder/nurses records
- Doctors/nurses should check feeding tube has been placed correctly either by A) x-ray, B) Injecting air into tube and listening for bubbling noises of gastric juice with a stethoscope over the stomach or C) Aspiration of gastric juices and testing with litmus (litmus paper should turn from blue to red if correctly in place). This will depend on hospital policy

Example of checklist for monitoring enteral tube feeding

- General patient's well being, ie tolerance to feed
- Weekly weight, to assess weight gain/loss and check fluid balance
- Daily urea and electrolytes (either on hospital computers or back of patient's medical notes or recorded in patient's medical notes)
- Daily fluid balance (in fluid charts in patient's bed-end folder), to monitor state of hydration
- Daily bowel movement (bed-end folder), to observe for diarrhoea or constipation
- Daily dietary intake (if applicable, in food intake charts in patient's bed-end folder or when possible by taking 24 hour diet history)
- Blood glucose (commonly in patient's observation chart with temperature and bowel action in bed-end folder). 4 hour initially for first two to three days
- Weekly anthropometry (eg weight, skin fold thickness etc)
- Other blood results and investigations as indicated (eg vitamin and mineral status, Liver Function tests and urinalysis)

Table 4.1 Complications associated with enteral tube feeding

Complication	Comments	Suggested remedies
Abnormal LFTs	Causes are multifactorial and relate to underlying disease or malnutrition	• Seldom clinically significant in patients without liver disease therefore rarely requires cessation of feed

Aspiration	Commonly caused by tube misplacement, delayed gastric emptying or poor gag reflex	• Check tube position (by x-ray or aspiration of gastric acid)
		  • Aspirate tube 4 - 6 hourly • Wide bore tube
		  • Elevate patient's head (to a minimum 30° angle)
		  • Reduce gastric motility using antiemetics (ref Table 6.10)
		  • If NG feeding, try naso-duodenal or naso-jejunal feeding if continual problem

Constipation	Patients may not be receiving sufficient fluids and/or fibre	• Extra fluid • Consider fibre containing feed • Appropriate enema, laxatives or bulking agents

Diarrhoea	Rapid feeding rates, bolus feeding and some antibiotics may cause diarrhoea
	Common in patients fed jejunally
	Check that this is not an 'overflow' from constipation
		• Send a stool sample for culture (to determine any microbial causes)
		  • Anti-diarrhoea agents (eg loperamide or codeine phosphate)
		  • Reduce feeding rate/ osmolarity • Reduce range of antibiotics if possible
		  • Consider fibre containing or lactose-free feed

Hyperglycaemia	Usually related to insulin resistance	• Insulin. Aim for continuous feeding to help maintain blood sugar control • Regular monitoring blood glucose, 4 hourly initially until blood sugars stabilise

Tube blockage	Continual feeding at very slow rates (eg 10mls/hr) may cause this and additions of medications and/or reconstituted feeds. Regular flushing of tube with sterile water should prevent this	• Flush tube with sterile water mixed with a pinch of sodium bicarbonate
		  or flush with pancreatic enzyme solution/diet cola/ cranberry or pineapple juice
		  • If administering drugs via feeding tube ensure they are finely crushed, in liquid form/syrup and that the tube is flushed well before and after drug administration

Tube withdrawal	Short term feeding tubes may be pulled out by patients by accident. Others may persistently refuse to keep them down	• If NG feeding, tape the tube securely to the patient's face • If persistently a problem consider long term feeding routes

Hyper/Hypo kalaemia, Natraemia, Phosphataemia	Renal/liver patients susceptible	• Adjust diet/or enteral feed accordingly, use of 'specialist feeds' as appropriate
		  • Regular monitoring blood biochemistry
		  • Sodium and/or Potassium supplements if v. low levels

Source: Adapted from Bowling and Silk (1994)

4

Patient name ....

Ward ....

Type of feed 1500mls standard 1kcal/ml

Type of tube ....

Date	Volume of feed/mls (total 1500mls)	Delivery rate (mls/hr)	Total feeding time (hrs)	Rest period (hrs)
Day 1	200	*50	4	
	300	75	4	
	500	100	5	
	500	125	4	7
Day 2	1500	125	12	12
Day 3 (established regimen)	1500	150	10	14

Flushing

Flush with .... ml sterile water at the beginning and end of feeding and between bottles/bags

Fluid regimes/flushes may be written within the feeding regimen as well.
(Giving set should be changed every 24 hours)

*If patient has had a prolonged period of starvation prior to feeding start feed rate at 25mls/hr.

NB: The above is intended as a guide only. Each patient should be individually assessed and reviewed regularly.

Fig 4.4 Example of a 1500 kcal Naso-Gastric pump starter feeding regimen

4

Patient name ....   Type of feed 2000mls standard 1kcal/ml

Ward ....   Type of tube ....

Date	Volume of feed/mls (total 2000mls)	Delivery rate (mls/hr)	Total feeding time (hrs)	Rest period (hrs)
Day 1	200	*50	4	
	300	75	4	
	500	100	5	
	500	125	4	7
Day 2	2000	125	16	8
Day 3 (established regimen)	2000	150	13.5	10.5

Flushing

Flush with .... ml sterile water at the beginning and end of feeding and between bottles/bags

Fluid regimes/flushes may be written within the feeding regimen as well.
(Giving set should be changed every 24 hours)

*If patient has had a prolonged period of starvation prior to feeding start feed rate at 25mls/hr.

NB: The above is intended as a guide only. Each patient should be individually assessed and reviewed regularly.

Fig 4.5 Example of a 2000 kcal Naso-Gastric pump starter feeding regimen

PEG starter regimen - Guidelines for feeding (first 24 hours)

Based on PEN Group guidelines

- 12 hours post insertion of PEG, flush tube with 50 mls of sterile water
- Three hours later, flush tube with another 50 mls of sterile water
- Three hours after that, flush tube with 50 mls of sterile water
- Commence starter feeding regimen (as a guide, start feeding rate at 25 mls/hr)

PEG maintenance

- Nurses should check surrounding skin of entry site of tube and clean daily (as it can become infected)
- Ensure giving set is changed daily
- Ensure feeding tube is flushed before and after feed administration

4

General enteral monitoring considerations

- Become familiar with your own hospitals tube feeding policies and protocols
- Assess how well the patient is tolerating the feed
- Be aware that feeding pumps may get switched off accidentally or to enable the patient to go for tests and/or physiotherapy etc
- Check to see if actual feed and feeding rate given to the patient matches your recommended tube feeding regimen
- Be prepared for patients who are non-compliant and repeatedly pull their short term feeding tubes out
- Be aware of problems associated with persuading patients and/or medical staff to allow tubes to be passed
- Check with nurses/doctors first, to establish how much the patient has been told before explaining tube feeding to them
- Always try to provide the easiest and most practical feeding regimen for both patient and nurses/carers to use
- Become familiar with feeding pump rates (ie intervals) and types of feeds used
- Individualise feeding regimens to each patient (eg some may require overnight, intermittent or continual feeding)

Home enteral nutrition

Expanding area involving:
- Multidisciplinary team approach
- Comprehensive patient education
- Delivery of feeding equipment and supplies
- Provision of follow-up nutrition care
- Psychosocial aspects

Elia (1994)

General Information:
- Most feeds are available on prescription
- Feeding equipment is not available on prescription (has to be financed by hospital or community budgets)
- Some nutrition companies will provide training and delivery of feeds and equipment/servicing of pumps at the patients homes
- Dietitians need approximately five days working notice for patients going home with tube feeds. This allows time to
  - contact the patient's GP to update them on their patient's care and ask if they will provide the feed on prescription,
  - time to educate the carers and inform the Nutrition Company of possible pumps required and deliveries
- UK dietitians should register their home enteral nutrition patients on the British Artificial Nutrition Survey (BANS) which is a home enteral feeding register to monitor aspects of care which vary in different Health Authorities
- Carers and relatives may initially need a 24 hour telephone helpline

Discontinuing tube feed

- Wean off gradually whilst encouraging, where appropriate, an increase in oral food intake (food charts to monitor intake)
- Try nutritional sip feeds, if meeting nutritional requirements is a problem
- Arrange follow up outpatient appointment/review by telephone if leaving hospital or review as appropriate

General information

- The Parenteral and Enteral Nutrition Group of The British Dietetic Association have produced student guidelines and a competency checklist for enteral and parenteral nutrition ([1+2] BDA, 1996)

- 'A Pocket Guide to Clinical Nutrition' is an excellent reference pocket book of clinical data primarily for nutritional support (Todorovic and Micklewright, 1997)

- If required, long term feeding tubes can be placed during a patient's surgical operation

- Nasoduodenal feeding is rarely used as patients with nausea/vomiting/aspiration usually require enteral tube feeding further down the gut, ie into the jejunum where these symptoms are less likely to persist

- Oro-Gastric feeding is also rarely used since it is uncomfortable for the patient as it can cause a 'dry' mouth and ulcerated lips

- Some ITU patients will automatically be tube or parenterally fed, due to their unconscious condition

4

References and further reading

Borlase B C (1994)
Enteral Nutrition, Chap and H Chapman and Hall series in Clinical Nutrition

Bowling T E and Silk (1994)
Enteral Feeding - problems and solutions, European Journal of Clinical Nutrition 48 (6) pp379-85

[1]**British Dietetic Association (BDA) (1996)**
Adult Enteral and Parenteral Nutrition: Guidelines for Dietitians in training, Parenteral and Enteral Nutrition Group of the British Dietetic Association

[2]**British Dietetic Association (BDA) (1996)**
Adult Enteral and Parenteral Nutrition: Guidelines for Dietitians in training, Competency checklist, Parenteral and Enteral Nutrition Group of the British Dietetic Association

Elia M (1994)
Home enteral nutrition:general aspects and a comparison between United States and Britain, Nutrition 10 (2) pp115-23

Enteral Nutrition (1990)
A Handbook for Dietitians & Health Professionals, Iowa State UP

Marks J M and Ponsky J L (1995)
Access routes for enteral nutrition, Gastroenterologist 3 (2) pp130-40

Mayhens S L and Thorn D (1995)
Enteral nutrition support:an overview, American Pharmacy NS 35 (2) pp47-59

Payne-James J J (1995)
Enteral Nutrition:Review, European Journal of Gastroenterology and Hepatology 7 (6) pp501-6

Rombeah J L, Calowell, Michael D, Rolandelli R H (1996)
Clinical Nutrition. V1: Enteral and Tube feeding, W B Saunders

Shikora S A (1996)
Nutrition Support: Theory and Therapeutics, Chap and Chapman and Hall Series in Clinical Nutrition

Skipper A (1997)
Dietitians Handbook of Enteral and Parenteral Nutrition, Americal Society for Parenteral and Enteral Nutrition (ASPEN) Publrs, USA

Thomas B (1994)
Manual of Dietetic Practice, 2nd Edition, Blackwell Scientific Publications

Todorovic V and Micklewright A (1997)
A Pocket Guide to Clinical Nutrition, 2nd Edition, Parenteral and Enteral Nutrition Group of the British Dietetic Association

4

Section 5

Parenteral Nutrition

Parenteral Nutrition (PN) -An overview

NB: Student and most basic grade dietitians would not be expected to manage PN patients. This section, however, gives a very general overview of what PN is. For further details consult The British Dietetics Association Guidelines and Competency checklist for Enteral and Parenteral Nutrition ([1 + 2] BDA, 1996).

Definition

- The delivery of nutrients directly into the circulatory system via a central venous catheter or via the peripheral veins also known as IV feeding and less commonly intravenous hyperalimentation (IVH)

- The term 'parenteral nutrition' (PN) is more accurate to use than 'total parenteral nutrition' since patients may be fed by a combination of both enteral and parenteral routes

Absolute indication

- Non Functioning Gut

Proven values

5

- Short Bowel Syndrome

- Enterocutaneous Fistula

- High Output Fistula

- Conditions requiring total bowel rest (eg post bowel surgery)

Examples of common PN fed patients

- Patients requiring total bowel rest (eg pre and/or post surgery)

- Patients with severe pancreatitis

- Inflammatory Bowel Disease (eg active Crohns Disease or Ulceratice Colitis)

- Patients with Enterocutaneous fistulas

- Radiation Enteritis

- Motility disorders, eg Scleroderma

- Chronic idiopathic intestinal pseudo-obstruction

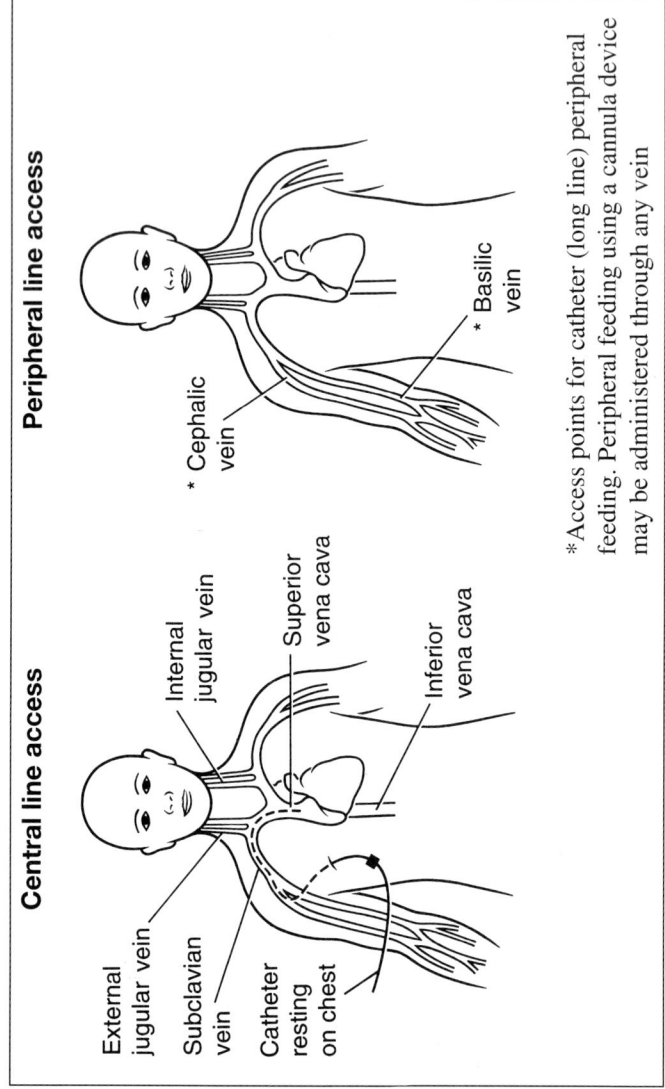

Fig 5.1: Parenteral nutrition - routes of administration

Central line access

External jugular vein

Internal jugular vein

Subclavian vein

Catheter resting on chest

Superior vena cava

Inferior vena cava

Peripheral line access

* Cephalic vein

* Basilic vein

*Access points for catheter (long line) peripheral feeding. Peripheral feeding using a cannula device may be administered through any vein

5

Routes of administration (refer fig 5.1)

Central line (For IV feeding required >10 - 14 days)

- Central vein cannulation (CVC) is currently the most commonly used route for administration (see Fig 5.1)
- A central feeding catheter is inserted aseptically via the subclavian vein into the superior vena cava
- The catheter is then tunnelled subcutaneously down into the chest (providing a flat surface for applying dressings)
- Common CVC access points include the subclavian vein, superior and inferior vena cava, internal and external jugular vein (see Fig 5.1)

Peripheral line (For IV feeding required <10 - 14 days)

- Peripheral vein canulation allows for access to the central system via a peripheral vein (see Fig 5.1)
- Peripheral feeding may be administered using a catheter or cannula device
- A catheter device (or 'long line') is more than 10 cm in length and is non-rigid when held horizontally
- Long lines are administered subcutaneously in to the basilic or cephalic vein
- As a patient is required to keep their arm (with the long line in-situ) outstretched, to allow full flow of the feed, this type of feeding is more suitable for immobile or unconscious patients
- Peripheral feeding using a cannula device may be administered through any vein
- Cannula devices are less than 10 cm in length and are rigid when held horizontally
- Using a cannula device may be more suitable for patients requiring peripheral feeding for 1 to 2 days as it is less intrusive than long line feeding
- Due to the osmolarity of 'normal' PN feeds and the viability of veins, peripheral feeding often results in a reduced total feed administration
- A typical Peripheral line feed regime is 9.4 g Nitrogen, 1400 - 1600 kcal (1000 kcals as lipid) and 3 litre volume

5

Initiating PN - assess:

- The degree of malnutrition (if applicable)
- The expected duration of non gut access and/or ability to absorb nutrients enterally
- The degree of metabolic stress
- The patient's prognosis
- Whether a standard pre-prepared bag or specially made up bag will be required eg for liver/renal patients or patients with a very high/low weight who would be either over or under fed with a standard bag.

Complications

Central line

- Central Vein Catheter (CVC) infection or CVC-related sepsis are most common
- Other insertion related complications include air embolism, arterial puncture, nerve injury and CV thrombosis

Peripheral line

- Peripheral Vein Thrombosis (PVT)

  Others include long term problems associated with over-feeding (eg fatty liver), nutritional deficiencies associated with underfeeding, mechanical and biochemical parameters

Guidelines for monitoring PN

- Clinical appearance
- Daily temperature
- Daily fluid balance
- Daily weights
- Serum glucose for whole period on PN - initially 4 hourly
- Urea and Electrolytes, liver function tests
- Other blood results as indicated (eg vitamin and mineral status)

- Twice weekly C-Reactive Protein, LFT's, bone calcium, phosphate and FBC
- Weekly trace elements and anthropometry
- Fortnightly copper, magnesium and zinc

Home PN

- Commonly given to patients with non-malignant diseases and gut failure incurred from other forms of treatment (eg surgery). Generally used for patients with an ischaemic gut
- Likely candidates include: short bowel syndrome patients, extensive Crohn's Disease, Radiation to the small intestine, refractory sprue, chronic adhesive obstruction or a diffuse motility gut disorder
- Delivery of home PN involves a multidisciplinary team approach consisting of: physicians, nurses, pharmacists, dietitians, gastroenterologists, surgeons and social workers (to assess suitability of patient and family for long term home PN) and NHS business managers to decide which Health Authority financially supports the feeding costs (Woods, 1995)

5

Additional information

- PN feeds are contained in aseptic, clear plastic bags (similar to IV fluid packaging) ready to hang from a drip stand
- PN bags contain a mixture of amino acids, glucose, lipids, electrolytes, trace elements and vitamins
- Commonly, Pharmacy Departments will provide 3 litre 'all in one' (AIO) bags containing the above
- Standard regimens or specially prepared bags can be made up depending on the individuals nutritional requirements
- Some bags may be covered by an additional silver bag on top to prevent the sunlight destabilising fat soluble vitamins
- Normally feeding pumps, similar to enteral feeding pumps, will administer the feed

References and further reading

[1]**British Dietetic Association (BDA) (1996)**
Adult Enteral and Parenteral Nutrition: Guidelines for Dietitians in training, Parenteral and Enteral Nutrition Group of the British Dietetic Association

[2]**British Dietetic Association (BDA) (1996)**
Adult Enteral and Parenteral Nutrition: Guidelines for Dietitians in training, Competency checklist, Parenteral and Enteral Nutrition Group of the British Dietetic Association

Dean R E (1990)
Training Manual for Total Parenteral Nutrition, Precept P USA

Finley T (1997)
Making sense of parenteral nutrition in adult patients, Nursing Times 82 (93) pp35-36

Grant A M, Todd E (1987)
Enteral and Parenteral Nutrition: A Clinical Handbook, Blackwell Scientific Publishers

Grant S and Todd E (1987)
Enteral and Parenteral Nutrition, 2nd Ed Blackwell Scientific Publications

Grimble G K; Payne-James J J; Rees R G P; Silk O B A (1990)
Nutrition Support - Theory and Practice, Medical Tribune U K Ltd

Heenan A L (1996)
Fluids used in total parenteral nutriton, Professional Nurse 11 (7) pp467-8, 470

Malone M (1995)
Parenteral Nutrition Support, UKCPA Clinical Pharmacy Practice Guide, No 9

Mattox T W; Bertch K E; Miratallo J M; Strausberg K M; Cuddy P G (1995)
Recent advances:parenteral nutrition support, Annals of Pharmacotherapy 29 (2) pp174-80

5

Meguid M M (1994)
Past, present and future of nutritional support, Nutrition 10 (5 Suppl) pp514-6

Nordenstorm J; Thorne A; (1994)
Benefits and complications of parenteral nutritional support, European Journal of Clinical Nutrition 48 (8) pp531-7

Payne-James J J; Grimble G K; Silk; (1995)
Artificial Nutrition Support in Clinical Practice, Edward Arnold

Rombean J L, Calowell, Michael D (1993)
Clinical Nutrition. V2: Parenteral Nutrition, W B Saunders

Shikora S A (1996)
Nutrition Support: Theory and Therapeutics, Chap and H Chapman and Hall series in Clinical Nutrition

Skipper A (1997)
Dietitian's Handbook of Enteral and Parenteral Nutrition, Americal Society for Parenteral and Enteral Nutrition (ASPEN) Publrs, USA

Taylors S and Goodinson-McLaren (1992)
Nutrition support:A team approach, Wolfe Publishing Ltd

Todorovic V and Micklewright A (1997)
A Pocket Guide to Clinical Nutrition. Parenteral and Enteral Nutrition Group of the British Dietetic Association

Wood S (1995)
Home parenteral nutrition quality criteria for clinical services and the supply of nutrient fluids and equipment, The British Association for Parenteral and Enteral Nutrition

5

5

Section 6

Drugs

Drugs

Notes

1. Examples of common drugs under each category are given according to 'approved name' ie chemical name, unless otherwise stated

2. Always consult the most recent edition of a British National Formulary (BNF) or Monthly Index of Medical Specialities (MIMS) for a full description of a drug. If unsure, consult a clinical pharmacist (drug information lines are available in hospitals)

3. Unless otherwise stated the following data has been compiled from September 1996 BNF

Table 6.1 - Oral Hypoglycaemics (over page)

Source: compiled with assistance from Mrs J Bowden (Pharmacist, The Royal Bournemouth Hospital), Mrs J Everett and Mrs P Miles (Diabetes Nurse Specialists, The Royal Bournemouth Hospital).

NB. Oral Hypoglycaemics should not be taken without food. Patients must be told how important this is. Hypos on tablets are very rare but if they do occur, are very dangerous, requiring hospital admission.

6

Diabetes

Table 6.1 - Oral Hypoglycaemics

Classification of Oral Hypoglycaemic	Common examples	Action	Side effects	Comments
Sulphonylureas	Chlorpropamide Glibenclamide *Gliclazide *Glipizide Gliquidone Tolazamide *Tolbutamide	• Stimulate the pancreas to release more insulin • Increases the body's sensitivity to insulin	• Generally mild and infrequent, include gastro-intestinal disturbances and headaches	• Most effective if taken half an hour before food • Can encourage weight gain therefore should not be first line of therapy for the overweight • Although there are several sulphonylureas there is no evidence for any differences in their effect
Biguanides	Metformin (Glucophage) Only biguanide available for prescription in the UK	Mechanism of action undetermined they may: • Decrease absorption of glucose from the intestine • Increase the uptake of glucose by the body tissues • Enhance the binding of insulin to its receptors making it more effective	• Can be nasty - nausea and/or vomiting, diarrhoea and risk of lactic acidosis in the elderly	• If maximum dose of sulphonylurea or biguanide is not sufficient, it is possible to add in another eg Tolbutamide 500mgs tds + Metformin 1g tds • Cause no risk of hypoglycaemia • Can help with weight loss as they prevent some of the uptake of CHO therefore most suitable for the overweight
Alpha Glucosidase Inhibitors	Acarbose (Glucobay) only product available	• Blocks the enzymes which break down large CHO molecules, eg starch into smaller molecules such as glucose • Only small molecules can be absorbed from the GI tract and so acarbose reduces CHO absorption	• May be troublesome, effect on GI tract	• Any glucose taken orally will still be absorbed • Must be taken with first mouthful of a meal • Acarbose may be used as first line therapy or added to other oral agents • Acarbose alone cannot cause hypoglycaemia but if used with other agents, sugar must not be used to treat hypo - use glucose

* shorter acting sulphonylureas used in the elderly

6

Diabetes (cont)

- Insulin is the hormone which allows glucose to be utilized by cells for the provision of energy

Table 6.2 Common insulins

Type of Insulin	Vials	Cartridges	Disposable Pens
Short acting			
Humulin S	✓	✓	✓ Humaject S
Actrapid	✓	✓ Actrapid Penfill	✓ Actrapid Pen
Pork Velosulin	✓	X	X
Human Velosulin	✓	X	X
Humalog	✓	✓	X
Intermediate acting			
Humulin I	✓	✓	✓ Humaject I
H. Insulatard	✓	✓ H. Insulatard Penfill	✓ H. Insulatard Pen
Pork Insulatard	✓	X	X
H. Monotard	✓	X	X
Long acting			
Ultratard	✓	X	X
Humulin Lente	✓	X	X
Humulin Zn	✓	X	X
Pork Lentard	✓	X	X
Mixtures			
10/90 Humulin M1	✓	✓	✓ Humaject MI
H. Mixtard 10	X	✓ H. Mixtard 10 Penfill	✓ H. Mixtard 10 Pen
20/80 Humulin M2	✓	✓	✓ Humaject M2
H. Mixtard 20	X	✓ H. Mixtard 20 Penfill	✓ H. Mixtard 20 Pen
30/70 Humulin M3	✓	✓	✓ Humaject M3
H. Mixtard 30	✓	✓ H. Mixtard 30 Penfill	✓ H. Mixtard 30 Pen
40/60 Humulin M4	✓	✓	✓ Humaject M4
H. Mixtard 40	X	✓ H Mixtard 40 Penfill	✓ H. Mixtard 40 Pen
50/50 Humulin M5	✓	✓	✓ Humaject M5
H. Mixtard 50	X	✓ H. Mixtard 50 Penfill	✓ H. Mixtard 50 Pen

Compiled by Mrs J Everett and Mrs P Miles (Diabetes Nurse Specialists, The Royal Bournemouth Hospital), reproduced with kind permission

NB Humulin Cartridges are licensed for BD pen. Mixtard Penfills are licensed for Novopen

6

Diarrhoea

- The first line of treatment for diarrhoea is to replace lost fluid and electrolytes (using oral rehydration preparations)

- Antibiotics can be used for treating Campylobacter Enteritis, invasive salmonellosis, shigellosis etc (ie systemic bacterial infections)

- Simple gastro-enteritis, even when a bacterial cause is suspected, rarely requires drug therapy since it usually clears up by itself

- If patient has diarrhoea request stool sample to be sent to microbiology to rule out any infectious causes before using antimotility drugs eg codeine, loperamide, co-phenotrope, morphine, to avoid risk of toxic megacolon

Table 6.3 - Common drugs used in the treatment of acute and chronic diarrhoea

Acute diarrhoea	Chronic diarrhoea
Kaolin (Adsorbent) Ispaghula Methylcellulose Sterculia Codeine Phosphate Co-phenotrope Loperamide Morphine Imodium	Mesalazine (eg for ulcerative colitis) Olsalazine (as above) Sulphasalazine (eg for ulcerative colitis or Crohn's Disease) Cholestyramine (eg for Crohn's, ileal resection, vagotomy, diabetic vagal neuropathy or radiation) Prednisolone (eg for ulcerative colitis or Crohn's) Sodium Cromoglycate (eg for food allergy)

NB Anti-motility drugs should not be used for the treatment of diarrhoea in children

6

Drugs that can cause diarrhoea

- The following drugs all contain sorbitol. Sorbitol taken in excess can cause diarrhoea (Greenwood 1989). The drugs listed below may cause diarrhoea as a side effect since they all contain sorbitol. However always eliminate other possible causes of the diarrhoea

Table 6.4 - Drugs which may cause diarrhoea

Drugs containing Sorbitol	
Aciclovir suspension	Indomethacin syrup
Alfacalcidol solution	Maalox suspension
Amitriptyline syrup	Metronidazole suspension
Atenolol syrup	Moduretic oral solution
Baclofen liquid	Mucaine suspension
Bumetanide liquid	Neomycin elixir
Carbamazepine syrup	Orphenadrine hydrochloride elixir
Chlormethiazole syrup	
Cimetidine suspension	Procyclidine syrup
Co-codamol dispersible tablets	Sodium valproate liquid
Diazepam syrup	Temazepam elixir
Ibuprofen syrup	Trazodone hydrochloride syrup
Imipramine syrup	

Compiled by Leighton Hospital Dietetic and Pharmacy Department. Reproduced with kind permission.

6

Laxatives

- Before laxatives are used it is important to be sure that the patient is constipated and the constipation isn't secondary to an underlying undiagnosed complaint
- It is also important for patients to understand that constipation is defined as the passage of hard stools less frequently than the patient's own normal pattern
- Excessive use of laxatives may lead to hypokalaemia and an atonic non-functioning colon
- A balanced diet with sufficient fibre and fluids as well as exercise is important in preventing constipation

Table 6.5 - Drugs used to relieve constipation

Laxative classification	Laxatives
Bulk-forming (increase faecal mass which stimulates peristalsis, may take 2 - 3 days to take full effect)	Trifyba (contains bran), Fybogel, Konsyl, Normacol, Isogel, Regulan, Celevac
Stimulant (acts as a stimulant agent. Increases intestinal motility and often causes abdo cramp, should seldom be needed)	Bisacodyl, Danthron, Docusate, Glycerol, Senna, Manevac, Sodium Picosulphate, Picolax
Faecal softeners (soften the stool)	Arachis Oil, Liquid Paraffin, Docusate
Osmotic laxative (act by retaining fluid in the bowel by osmosis)	Lactulose, Magnesium Hydroxide Mixture

Table 6.6 - Drugs that can cause constipation

Drug classification	
Aluminium containing antacids	Diuretics
Anticholinergics (including tricyclics, phenothiazines)	Iron preparations
Antihistamines	Levodopa (in Sinemet and Madopar)
Calcium channel blockers (eg Verapamil)	MAOIs
Clonidine	Opiates (including co-proxamol/ co-dydramol, morphine)

Compiled by The Royal Bournemouth Hospital Pharmacy Department. Reproduced with kind permission

6

Diuretics

- A drug that increases the volume of urine produced by promoting the excretion of salts and water from the kidney
- Diuretics are used to reduce oedema due to salt and water retention in disorders of the heart, kidneys or lungs
- Some diuretics are used in conjunction with other drugs to reduce blood pressure (refer table 6.7)

Table 6.7 - Common drug examples of diuretics

Diuretic classification	Diuretics
Thiazide and related (relieve oedema due to heart failure)	Bendrofluazide, Chlorothiazide, Chlorthalidone, Cyclopenthiazide, Hydrochlorothiazide, Indapamide, Mefruside, Metolazone, Xipamide
Loop (for patients with pulmonary oedema due to left ventricular failure)	Frusemide, Bumetanide
Potassium sparing (causes retention of potassium)	Amiloride, Triamterene, Spironolactone
Carbonic Anhydrase Inhibitors (weak diuretic used in glaucoma)	Acetazolamide, Dichlorphenamide
Diuretics with potassium (for patients requiring potassium supplementation)	Burinex K, Diumide-K, Lasikal, Lasix + K, Neo-NaClex-K

Table 6.8 - Lipid lowering drugs

Lipid lowering drugs		
Cholestyramine	Gemfibrozil	Nicotinic Acid
Colestipol	Fluvastatin	Omega-3 Marine-Triglycerides
Bezafibrate	Pravastatin	Probucol
Ciprofibrate	Simvastatin	
Fenofibrate	Acipimox	

6

Table 6.9 - Drug-nutrient interactions

Drug classification	Comments
Acitretin	Fatty foods increase the absorption of acitretin
Anticoagulants	Foods rich in Vitamin K can reduce the effects of warfarin
Ciprofloxacin	Dairy products reduce bioavailability of ciprofloxacin and norfloxacin
Cyclosporin	Food, milk and grapefruit juice can increase the bioavailability of cyclosporin
Hydralazine	Food can significantly reduce the bioavailability and peak serum levels of hydralazine
Isoniazid	Isoniazid with histamine rich foods (eg cheese, tuna) may cause a flushing reaction with headache, difficulty in breathing, nausea and tachycardia
MAOI's	Patients taking MAOI's can suffer a serious hypertensive reaction if they consume tyramine rich foods such as cheese and beer
Phenytoin	A very marked reduction in phenytoin absorption has been seen when given with enteral feeds given via a naso-gastric tube. Enteral tube feeds should be stopped two hours before administration of Phenytoin and restarted 2 hours post administration of Phenytoin
Rifampicin	Food delays and reduces the absorption of rifampicin from the gut
Sodium Clodronate and Disodium Etidronate	Absorption is reduced by antacids, iron preparations, calcium supplements, milk and food containing calcium, magnesium and aluminium
Tetracyclines, eg oxytetracycline	Absorption is markedly reduced if allowed to come into contact with milk or other dairy products

Compiled by The Royal Bournemouth Hospital Pharmacy Department.
Reproduced with kind permission

6

Table 6.10 - Common drug examples of antiemetics (for nausea and vomiting)

Antiemetic	
Metoclopramide	Methotrimeprazine
Prochlorperazine	Droperidol
Cyclizine	Haloperidol
Domperidone	Ondansetron

NB In all cases antiemetics should only be prescribed once the cause of vomiting is known

Table 6.11 - Common drug examples of appetite stimulants and suppressants

Appetite stimulants	Appetite suppressants
Gentian Mixture, Acid BP, Gentian Mixture, Alkaline BP (eg Effico, Labiton and Metatone) Steroids Alcohol	Bulk forming Drugs eg Celevac Centrally acting appetite suppressants eg *Dexfenfluramine(Adifax), *Fenfluramine (Ponderax), Phenteramine (Duromine)

NB Appetite suppressants are not a means of treating obesity in the long term. They can play only a limited role and should never be used as the sole source of treatment.

* Withdrawn from the market as from September 1997

6

References and further reading

Kirk J K (1995)
Significant drug-nutrient interactions, American Family Physcian 51 (5) pp1175-82

British National Formulary (September 1996)
British Medical Association and the Royal Pharmaceutical Society of Great Britain, Number 31

Greenwood J (1989)
Sugar content of liquid prescription medicines, The Pharmaceutical Journal Part 6 (243) pp243.

Monthly Index of Medical Specialities (September 1997)
Haymarket Medical Ltd

Thomas J A (1995)
Drug-nutrient interactions, Nutrition Reviews 53 (10) pp271-82

6

Section 7

Product Information

Product Information (for nutritional supplements)

Product information notes

- Products are listed in alphabetical order by product name, within appropriate category (refer below)

- Nutritional composition is given per total volume/weight of each product. Where more than one volume/weight exists per product, nutritional composition for the lowest measure available is given

- Occasionally, slight differences in nutritional composition occur between different flavours of the same product. In this instance nutritional composition has been given for the most predominant similar values amongst the flavours (usually only flavours such as chocolate raise energy and fat values slightly)

- Feeds designed specifically for paediatrics and metabolic disorders have been omitted

- Some feeds not available on prescription may be available on prescription by a named patient system. For up-to-date information of nutritional supplements and prices consult a current BNF or MIMS. Alternatively contact nutrition company information office lines (refer page 138)

- Compositional data was compiled from The British Dietetic Association's Advisor Tube and Sip Feed Chart (Feb 1995), The British National Formulary (Sept 1995) and Manufacturers Nutrition Services and/or published literature

- All product data correct to the best of the authors knowledge for Sept 1997

Definition of supplement categories

Sip feed (Nutritional Supplements)

7

Products intended to be sipped orally. Most are nutritionally complete, presented as a tetra brick with attached straw.

Tube feed

Any product intended for use as a tube feed presented in a can, soft pouch/ready to hang, glass or plastic bottle. Most are nutritionally complete. All feeds in this section may also be taken orally but are classed under this category because they are nearly always administered by an enteral feeding tube.

Energy supplement

Any product derived from a carbohydrate or fat source (or both) either as a powder or liquid, primarily high in energy only.

Protein supplement

Product specifically high in protein but low in most other nutrients.

Thickeners

Any product in powder form used specifically to thicken food and fluids.

Fortified milk shakes/puddings/soups

Ready to eat/drink or powder form, fortified with energy, protein and some vitamins and minerals. Not nutritionally complete. Some are not available on prescription.

Product information key

Flavours

ap	- apple	man	- mandarin
asp	- asparagus	mel	- melon
apr	- apricot	moc	- mocha
ban	- banana	mush	- mushroom
bla	- blackcurrant	mus	- muesli
but	- butterscotch	n	- neutral
cap	- cappuccino	nut	- nut
car	- caramel	or	- orange
che	- cherry	org	- original
choc	- chocolate	pe	- peach
chocmt	- chocolate mint	p+o	- peach and orange
chi	- chicken	p+r	- peach and raspberry
cof	- coffee	pine	- pineapple
d+b	- dandelion and burdock	p+l	- potato and leek
eg	- egg nog	ras	- raspberry
ff	- fruits of forest forest fruits	str	- strawberry
		sf	- summer fruits
fp	- fruit punch	tf	- tropical fruits
gr	- grapefruit	tof	- toffee
l+l	- lemon and lime	van	- vanilla
lem	- lemon	ve	- vegetable, vegetable cream

7

Presentations

Bar	- Bar		PB	- Plastic bottle
Can	- Can		Pot	- Pot
Drum	- Drum		Sachet	- Sachet
Gable	- Gable top carton		SP	- Soft pouch/semi rigid
GB	- Glass bottle		Tetra	- Tetra brick carton
Jar	- Jar		Tub	- Tub

Abbreviations (other)

Manufac	- Manufacturers		Present	- Presentation
Volume/wt	- Volume/weight		Kcal	- Kilocalories
ACBS approv	- ACBS approved		Kj	- Kilojoules
	(ie available on		Na	- Sodium
	prescription)		K	- Potassium

Manufacturers

Boots	- Boots
Cow & Gate	- Cow and Gate, a Division of Nutricia Ltd
Fresenius	- Fresenius Ltd
Heinz	- H J Heinz Co. Ltd
MJ	- Mead Johnson
NCN	- Nestlé Clinical Nutrition, a Division of Nestlé (formally Clintec Nutrition Ltd)
Nestlé	- Nestlé UK Ltd
Novartis	- Novartis Nutrition
NCC	- Nutricia Clinical Care, a Division of Nutricia Ltd
Ross	- Ross Products, a Division of Abbott Laboratories Ltd
SB	- Smith Kline Beecham
SH	- Sutherland Health
SHS	- Scientific Hospital Supplies
VF	- Vitaflo
UN	- Unigreg Ltd

7

Table 7.1 - Sip feeds (milk based)

Product	Manufac	Present	Volume/ Wt	ACBS Approv	Flavours	Energy kcal (KJ)	Protein g	Na mmol	K mmol	Comments
Complan	Heinz	Tetra	230ml	Pending	str,van,choc	250 (1050)	8.7	6.0	11.7	Nutritionally complete ready to drink milk tasting sip feed containing skimmed milk and lactose
Ensure Plus	Ross	Tetra	200ml	*	cof,car,bla, ban,choc,or, van,str,ras,ff	300 (1260)	12.5	10.43	9.41	High energy/low volume milk tasting sip feed. 1.5 kcal/ml
Entera	Fresenius	Tetra	200ml	*	van,str, choc+mt, bla,but,pine, or,ban,n,yg	300 (1260)	11.3	7.0	9.0	High energy/low volume milk tasting sip feed. 1.25 kcal/ml
Fortifresh	NCC	Tetra	200ml	Pending	ras,bla,man	310 (1298)	13	3.74	7.7	Nutritionally complete, energy dense, yoghurt tasting sip feed. Not suitable for vegetarians. 1.55 kcal/ml
Fortimel	NCC	Tetra	200ml	*	str,ff,van	200 (840)	19.4	4.34	10.26	High protein milk tasting sip feed. Suitable for patients on Na restriction. 1 kcal/ml
Fortisip	NCC	Tetra	200ml	*	ban,or,str,tf,tof,n van,mush,chi, choc	300 (1270)	10	6.88	7.5	High energy milk tasting/low volume sip feed. 1.5 kcal/ml. Chicken and mushroom flavours contain 14.2mmol Na per 200ml
Fresubin	Fresenius	Tetra	200ml	*	van,nut,pe, choc,moc,bla	200 (840)	7.6	6.6	6.4	High energy milk tasting sip feed. Suitable for patients on a K restriction. 1.0 kcal/ml
Fresubin Plus F	Fresenius	Tetra	200ml	*	mus	200 (840)	7.6	6.6	6.4	1g Fibre/100 ml. 1 kcal/ml

Table 7.1 - Sip feeds (milk based) continued

Product	Manufac	Present	Volume/ Wt	ACBS Approv	Flavours	Energy kcal (KJ)	Protein g	Na mmol	K mmol	Comments
Resource Shake	Novartis	Gable	175ml		van,choc,str	302 (1269)	9.0	3.2	4.7	High energy milk tasting microsip feed based on fresh milk. 1.7 kcal/ml. Initially frozen but then thawed when ready to use
Sno-Pro	SHS	Tetra	200ml	*	n	134 (560)	0.44	<6.6	<2.6	Low protein milk replacer. Also low in pheny-lalanine (25 mg/unit). Suitable for PKU, inborn areas of metabolism and renal patients. Not a sip feed. Not nutritionally complete
Tonexis	NCN	Tetra	200ml	*	choc,van, ff,cof	200 (840)	7.5	3.0	6.7 - 7.7	Milk tasting sip feed. 1 kcal/ml
Tonexis 1.5	NCN	Tetra	200ml	*	van,apr,sf, ban,choc	300 (1260)	11.2	7.0	6.2	High energy milk tasting sip feed 1.5 kcal/ml
Tonexis HP	NCN	Tetra	200ml	*	str,van,car chocnt,pe,	200 (840)	15	6.0	7.2 - 8.7	High protein. low volume milk tasting sip feed. 1 kcal/ml

7

Table 7.1 - Sip feeds (milk based) continued

Product	Manufac	Present	Volume/ Wt	ACBS Approv	Flavours	Energy kcal (KJ)	Protein g	Na mmol	K mmol	Comments

7

Teble 7.2 - Sip feeds (fruit flavoured)

Product	Manufac	Present	Volume/ Wt	ACBS Approv	Flavours	Energy kcal (KJ)	Protein g	Na mmol	K mmol	Comments
Elemental 028 Extra Liquid	SHS	Tetra	250ml	*	or+pine, gr,sf	215 (896)	6.2	6.8	6	Amino acid based fruit drink tasting supplement for patients with short bowel syndrome after intestinal resection. Crohn's disease and intractable malabsorption, eg HIV and Bowel Fistula
Enlive	Ross	Tetra	240ml	*	or,ap, l+l, pine,str,pe, gr,fp	300 (1274)	9.6	3.13	32.6	Fruit drink tasting supplement 1.25 kcal/ml
Fortijuce	NCC	Tetra	200ml	*	p+o,l+l,sf, bla,apr,pine, d+b	250 (1046)	8	1.04	1.3	Fruit drink tasting sip feed 1.25 kcal/ml
Provide	Fresenius	Tetra	250ml	*	tf,ap,l+l,bla	150 (630)	9	2.93	0.96	Higher in protein, fruit drink tasting sip feed. Suitable for patients with milk intolerance 0.6 kcal/ml
Provide Xtra	Fresenius	Tetra	200ml	*	l+l,ap,bla, mel,che, or+pine	250 (1046)	7.5	2.4	1.4	Higher in protein, fruit tasting sip feed. Suitable for patients with milk intolerance 1.25 kcal/ml

7

Table 7.2 - Sip feeds (fruit flavoured) continued

Product	Manufac	Present	Volume/ Wt	ACBS Approv	Flavours	Energy kcal (KJ)	Protein g	Na mmol	K mmol	Comments

7

Table 7.3 - Tube feeds (Whole Protein)

Product	Manufac	Present	Volume/ Wt	ACBS Approv	Flavours	Energy kcal (KJ)	Protein g	Na mmol	K mmol	Comments
Advera	Ross	Can	237 ml	*	choc.or	299 (1262)	14.2	10.43	15.38	Formulated to meet the nutritional needs of HIV/AIDS patients. 1.3 kcal/ml
AlitraQ	Ross	Sachet	76 g		n	300 (1282)	15.8	13.04	9.23	Nutritional values per 300 ml (reconstituted as directed) Glutamine-enriched enteral feed to meet the needs of critically ill patients. 1 kcal/ml
Clinifeed 1S0	NCN	Can	375 ml	*	van	400 (1575)	10.5	5.7	14.4	Milk free, low in Na and Protein. 1 kcal/ml
Clinifeed 1.0	NCN	DF	500 ml 1000 ml	* *	n	500 (2100) 1000 (4200)	19	13	15	Hypotonic milk free 1 kcal/ml
Clinifeed 1.5	NCN	DF	500 ml 1000 ml	* *	n	750 (3200) 1500 (6400)	28	24	22	High energy/low volume feed 1.5 kcal/ml
Clinifeed Fibre	NCN	DF	500 ml 1000 ml	* *	n	500 (2100) 1000 (4200)	19	13	14	Fibre enriched standard feed 1 kcal/ml
Enrich	Ross	Can	250ml	*	van,choc	256 (1079)	9.4	8.7	9.49	Sip or tube feed. 1.4g fibre/100ml. 1 kcal/ml
Ensure	Ross	Can	250ml	*	van,choc, msuh.cof, eg, chi,nut,asp	251 (1057)	10.0	9.57	9.49	Sip or tube feed. 1 kcal/ml
Ensure Plus	Ross	Can GB PB	250ml 500ml 1l	* * *	n n n	375 (1578)	15.6	13.1	11.6	High energy/low volume feed 1.5 kcal/ml

7

Table 7.3 - Tube feeds (Whole Protein) continued

Product	Manufac	Present	Volume/ Wt	ACBS Approv	Flavours	Energy kcal (KJ)	Protein g	Na mmol	K mmol	Comments
Entera	Fresenius	SP	500ml	*	n	750 (3138)	28	21.5	15.9	High energy/low volume feed. 1.5 kcal/ml
Fresubin	Fresenius	SP	500ml 1l	*	pe,van,n, nut	500 (2100)	19	16.6	16	Nutritionally complete. 1 kcal/ml
Fresubin 750 MCT	Fresenius	SP	500ml	*	van	750 (3150)	37.5	26	30	High in protein, energy and MCT. 1.5 kcal/ml
Fresubin Isofibre	Fresenius	SP	500ml 1l	*	n	500 (2100)	19	29	26	Isotonic, 1.5g fibre/100ml. 1 kcal/ml
Generaid Plus	SHS	Tub	400g	*	n	1852 (7776)	44	12	48	Orange flavoured free amino acid mixture high in BCAA. Used in the treatment of hepatic failure for sip or tube feeding
Introlite	Ross	PB	1l		n	530 (2250)	22	39.13	40.26	Low osmolarity feed with reduced energy, 0.53 kcal/ml and protein. 2.2g/100ml. for patients who cannot tolerate full strength formulas
Jevity	Ross	GB PB PB	500ml 1l 1.5l	* * *	n n	500 (2103)	20	19.13	18.97	Fibre-enriched isotonic feed. 1.4g fibre/ 100 ml. kcal/ml
Nepro	Ross	Can	237ml	*	n	475 (1991)	16.6	8.26	6.38	For renal patients on dialysis. Low electrolyte sip or tube feed. 2 kcal/ml

Table 7.3 - Tube feeds (Whole Protein) continued

Product	Manufac	Present	Volume/ Wt	Flavours	ACBS Approv	Energy kcal (KJ)	Protein g	Na mmol	K mmol	Comments
Nutrison concentrated LE	NCC	GB SP	500ml 500ml	n n		1000 (4200)	37.5	21.5	1g	Energy dense feed for patients requiring restricted fluid and electrolyte intakes. 2kcal/ml, 7.5g protein/100ml
Nutrison Energy	NCC	GB PB SP	5ooml 1l 1l	n n n	* * *	750 (3150)	30	17.5	17.5	High energy, low volume feed. 1.5 kcal/ml
Nutrison Fibre	NCC	GB PB SP	500 ml 1l 1l	n n n	* * *	500 (2100)	20	17.5	17.5	1.5g fibre/100ml. 1kcal/nl
Nutrison Low Protein Mineral	NCC	GB SP	500ml 500ml	n n		1000 (4200)	20	21.5	19	Low protein, energy dense feed. failure. For use in renal/liver 2 kcal/ml
Nutrison Low Na	NCC	GB SP	500ml 1000ml	n n		500 (2100)	20	5.5	17.5	Low in Na (1.1mmol/100ml) 1kcal/ml
Nutrison Soya	NCC	GB PB SP	500ml 1l 1l	n n n	* * *	500 (2092)	20	17.5	17.5	Isotonic, milk free feed. 1.kcal/ml
Nutrison Standard	NCC	GB PB SP	500ml 1l 1l	n n n	* * *	500 (2100)	20	17.5	17.5	Isotonic feed. 1.kcal/ml
Osmolite	Ross	Can GB PB PB	250ml 500ml 1l 1.5	n n n	* * * *	252 (1061)	10	9.56	9.48	Isotonic feed. 1 kcal/ml

7

89

Table 7.3 - Tube feeds (Whole Protein) continued

Product	Manufac	Present	Volume/ Wt	ACBS Approv	Flavours	Energy kcal (KJ)	Protein g	Na mmol	K mmol	Comments
Pre-Nutrison	NCC	GB SP	500ml 1l		n n	250 (1046)	10	8.5	8.5	Hypotonic, half strength feed for patients who cannot tolerate full strength feeds or require extra fluid. 0.5 kcal/ml
Pulmocare	Ross	Can GB	250ml 1l		n n	375 (1565)	15.63	1413	11.15	High fat, low CHO feed, designed for patients with compromised respiratory function. 1.5 kcal/ml
Suplena	Ross	Can	237ml	*	n	476 (1994)	7.1	8.26	6.82	For patients with protein, fluid and electrolyte restrictions. Sip or tube feed. 1 kcal/ml
Two Cal HN	Ross	Can	237ml	*	n	479 (2010)	19.8	13.48	14.72	For catabolic patients following severe trauma. 2 kcal/ml

Table 7.3 - Tube feeds (Whole Protein) continued

Product	Manufac	Present	Volume/ Wt	ACBS Approv	Flavours	Energy kcal (KJ)	Protein g	Na mmol	K mmol	Comments

7

Table 7.4 - Tube feeds (Elemental and semi-elemental)

Product	Manufac	Present	Volume/ Wt	ACBS Approv	Flavours	Energy kcal (KJ)	Protein g	Na mmol	K mmol	Comments
Dialamine	SHS	Tub	200g	*	or	720 (3060)	50	<0.8	<0.4	Orange flavoured free amino acid mixture, designed to give optimum essential amino acid intake. For oral or tube feeding. For advanced chronic renal failure. Not nutritionally complete.
Elemental 028	SHS	Sachet	100g	*	or,n	388 (1640)	10	10.8	11.9	High osmolarity, hypoallergenic, low fat. Amino acid based
EO28 Extra	SHS	Sachet	100g	*	or,n	427 (1793)	12.5	13.3	11.9	Hypoallergenic, elemental, increased N, fat and energy, glutamine and arginine
Emsogen	SHS	Sachet	100g	*	or,n	418 (1754)	12.5	13	11.9	Most fat as MCT (83%)
Flexical	MJ	Tub	454g	*	n	1997 (8355)	44.9	30.41	64.01	Semi-elemental
Hepatamine	SHS	Tub	60g		or	216 (918)	15	0.24	0.18	For use in hepatic failure. Supplement added to tube feed. Contains branched chain amino acids
Liquisorbon MCT	NCC	GB	500ml	*						MCT tube feed, gluten free. For patients with short bowel syndrome and fat malabsorption
Survimed OPD	Fresenius	SP GB	500ml 500ml	*	n	500 (2100)	22.5	29	20	MCT is major fat source. 1 kcal/ml Semi-elemental
MCT Pepdite 2+	SHS	Can	400g	*	n	1812 (7616)	55.2	36.4	52.8	Most fat as MCT. Contains peptides and free amino acids
Pepdite 2+	SHS	Can	400g	*	n	1756 (7376)	55.2	36.4	52.8	For sip or tube feeding
Peptamen	NCN	Can	250ml	*	van,n	250 (1045)	10	5.45	8.0	70% of fat as MCT, hypotonic. 1 kcal/ml

Table 7.4 - Tube feeds (Elemental and semi-elemental) continued

Product	Manufac	Present	Volume/ Wt	ACBS Approv	Flavours	Energy kcal (KJ)	Protein g	Na mmol	K mmol	Comments
Peptamen Flavoured	NCN	Sachets	24x4g	*	choc,str, van,lem,cap	12 - 15 (62)	0.14			Added to Peptamen to add flavour
Pepti-2000 LF (liquid)	NCC	GB SP	500ml 1l	* *	n	500 (2100)	20	17.5	18	Semi-elemental. low fat. 1 kcal/ml
Pepti 2000 LF(powder)	NCC	Sachet	126g	*		500 (2100)	20	10.2	18.1	Semi-elemental. low fat. Reconstituted for patients with inflammatory bowel disease and malabsorption
Perative	Ross	Can PB	237ml 1l	* *	n n	310 (1308)	15.8	10.87	10.51	Semi-elemental. 1.3 kcal/ml
Reabilan	NCN	Can SP	375ml 500ml	* *	n n	375 (1575)	12	11	13	Semi-elemental. 1 kcal/ml

7

Table 7.5 - Fortified milk shakes (Powders)

Product	Manufac	Present	Volume/ Wt	ACBS Approv	Flavours	Energy kcal (KJ)	Protein g	Na mmol	K mmol	Comments
Build Up	Nestlé NCN	Sachet + box	38g x 4 266g		l+l,str,van, choc.n.chi, p+l,mush	350 (1490) 330 (1390) 275 (1155)	23.1 18.2 18.5	16.3 0.4 (g) 0.4 (g)	28.6 20.76 21.53	Per 100g dry powder. Approximate figures variations exist between some varieties Per 38g sachet made up with 284 ml (1/2 pint) whole milk Per 38g sachet made up with 284 ml (1/2 pint) semi-skimmed milk
Complan	Heinz	sachet +Jar + Box	57g x 4 450g 55g		ban,choc, org, p+r, str, van, ve, chi	251 (1057)	8.8			Per 57g sachet made up with 200 mls water. Can also be reconstituted with milk. Vegetable and chicken flavours higher in sodium (29 mmol) and lower in potassium (6.2 mmol) compared to other flavours.
Scandi-shake	SHS	Sachet	85g	*	van,str choc	437 (1831) 437 (1831) 514 (2153) 598 (2505)	4 4 4.7 11.7	3.9 5.2 4.6 9.7	6.7 15.9 7.8 15.3	Per 85g powdered sachet (2 kcal/ml when made up with whole milk). High energy milkshake Per 100g powdered product Per 1 serving (85g powder and 240 ml whole milk
Recovery	Boots	Sachet +Jar	55g x 4 500g		choc.str.org	384 (1612) 336 (1408)	19 16	1.3 1.3	26.2 21.48	Per 100g dry powder Per 55g serving made with whole milk

+Jar/Box presentations available in neutral or original flavours only.

NB All the above milk shakes are nutritionally incomplete and therefore are not suitable as a sole source of nutrition for prolonged periods of time. They may also be unsuitable for patients on a low fat diet or for those who have a milk intolerance.

7

Table 7.5 - Fortified milk shakes (Powders) continued

Product	Manufac	Present	Volume/ Wt	ACBS Approv	Flavours	Energy kcal (KJ)	Protein g	Na mmol	K mmol	Comments

7

Table 7.6 - Fortified puddings

Product	Manufac	Present	Volume/ Wt	ACBS Approv	Flavours	Energy kcal (KJ)	Protein g	Na mmol	K mmol	Comments
Emelis	NCN	Pot	125g	*	pe,van, choc,car	153 (640)	11.3	7.06	9.93	Semi-solid milk tasting pudding, for patients with dysphagia
Formance	Ross	Can	142g	*	van,choc, but	250 (1052)	6.8	10.43	8.46	As above
Forti-pudding	NCC	Tub	150g	*	choc,cof, van	198 (840)	15.3	3.3	6.3	Semi-solid, high protein milk tasting pudding, for patients with dysphagia
Maxisorb	SHS	Sachets	30g	*	choc,str,van	138 (579)	12	1.8	4.1	High protein dessert mix

Table 7.7 - Fortified soups

Product	Manufac	Present	Volume/ Wt	ACBS Approv	Flavours	Energy kcal (KJ)	Protein g	Na mmol	K mmol	Comments
Build up	NCN	Sachets	40g		chi.mush, p+l	380-390 (1615 - 1655)	20.5	78	23	Mix with water. P+l lowest in energy, high in Na, negligible fibre. Nor nutritionally complete. Approximate figures. Variations exist between some varieties
Complan	Heinz	Sachets	57g		chi.ve	434 (1815)	21.0	78	23	Mix with water. High in Na. Not nutritionally complete

Table 7.8 - Energy supplements

Product	Manufac	Present	Volume/ Wt	ACBS Approv	Flavours	Energy kcal (KJ)	Comments
Calogen	SHS	GB	250ml 1l	* *	but,n	1125 (4625)	LCT fat emulsion. 4.5 kcal/ml
Caloreen	NCN	Tub	250g	*	n	1000 (4185)	Glucose polymer. 1.6 kcal/g
Calsip	Fresenius	Tetra	200ml	*	ap,pine.n	400 (1680)	High energy. low volume liquid CHO supplement. 2 kcal/ml
Duobar	SHS	Bar	100g	*	str,van	602 (2506)	Fat and CHO in solid form, protein free
Duocal Liquid	SHS	GB	250ml 1l	* *	n n	375 (1570)	Fat and glucose polymer, protein free. 1.6 kcal/ml
Duocal Super Soluble	SHS	Tub	400g	*	n	1968 (8244)	Fat and glucose polymer, protein free. 4.9 kcal/ml
Hycal	SB	GB	171ml	*	lem,bla, ras,or,ap	419 (1782)	Glucose polymer solution. 4.2 kcal/ml
Liquigen	SHS	GB	250ml 1l	* *	n	1125 (4625)	MCT fat emulsion. 4 kcal/ml
Maxijul Liquid	SHS	Tetra	200ml	*	n,bla,l+l,or	400 (1700)	Glucose polymer liquid. 2 kcal/ml
Maxijul LE	SHS	Can Tub	200g 2kg	* *	n	760 (3230)	Glucose polymer, low in electrolytes. 3.8 kcal/ml
Maxijul Super Soluble	SHS	Sachet Tub Drum	132g 200g 2.5kg 25kg	* * * *	n	502 (2132)	Glucose polymer. 3.8 kcal/ml
MCT Duocal	SHS	Tub	400g		n	1944 (8168)	Mostly MCT fat and glucose polymer (83%). 5 kcal/g

Table 7.8 - Energy Supplements continued

Product	Manufac	Present	Volume/ Wt	ACBS Approv	Flavours	Energy kcal (KJ)	Comments
MCT Oil	SHS	GB	500ml	*	n	4275 (17275)	MCT Oil. 8.5 kcal/ml
MCT Oil	MJ	GB	950ml		n		MCT Oil kcal/ml
Polycal Powder	NCC	Tub	400g	*	n	1520 (6460)	Glucose polymer powder. 3.8 kcal/ml
Polycal Liquid	NCC	GB	200ml	*	ap,bla,lem,or,n	500 (2100)	Glucose polymer solution. 2.5 kcal/ml
Polycose	Ross	Tub	350g	*	n	1316 (5264)	Glucose polymer. 3.8 kcal/ml
Vitajoule	VF	Sachet	130g		n	494 (2093)	Glucose polymer. 3.8 kcal/ml
		Tub	500g		n		
			2.5kg		n		
			25kg		n		

Table 7.8 - Energy supplements continued

Product	Manufac	Present	Volume/ Wt	ACBS Approv	Flavours	Energy kcal (KJ)	Comments

7

Table 7.9 - Protein supplements

Product	Manufac	Present	Volume/ Wt	ACBS Approv	Flavours	Protein g	Comments
Casilan 90	Heinz	Tub	250g	*	n	225	0.9g protein/g
Forceval Protein	UG	Sachet Tub	15g 300g	* *	str,van,n,choc	8.25 0.55	0.5g protein/g Calcium caseinate with 25 vitamins and minerals
Maxipro Super Soluble HBV	SHS	Tub	200g 1kg	* *	n	160	Whey protein powder concentrate supplemented with AA's For use in hypoproteinaemia 0.8g Protein/g
Promod	Ross	Tub	275g	*	n	206	Concentrated source of high quality protein (whey and lecithin) 0.75g protein/g
Prosource	Fresenius	Tub	275g		n	220	1.25g protein/g. Contains whey protein concentrate and calcium caseinate
Protifar	NCC	Tub	225g	*	n	199.1	Concentrated milk powder protein. 0.8g Protein/g
Vitapro	VF	Tub	250g 1kg	* *	n n	187.5	Milk protein 0.75 Protein/g

7

Table 7.10 - Thickeners

Product	Manufac	Present	Volume/Wt	ACBS Approv	Flavours	Comments
Nestargel	Nestlé	Tub	125g	*	n	Carob seed flour and Calcium Lactate. A natural thickening agent indicated for use in the dietary management of infantile or adult vomiting, including nausea and vomiting during pregnancy
Nutrilis	NCC	Tub Sachet	225g 8g		n	Modifiedmaize starch
Resource thicken up	Novartis	Tub	227g		n	Modified food starch indicated for any patient requiring thickening of liquid or food dysphagia. Contains vitamins and minerals but not nutritionally complete
Thick and Easy	Fresenius	Tub	225g 4.5kg	* *	n	Modified maize starch and maltodextrin
Thixo-D	SH	Tub	375g	*	n	Modified maize starch
Thixo-D Drink Mixes	SH	Tub	560g		ban,choc, or,str	High energy, thickened drinks
Thixo-D Cal-Free	SH	Tub	30g		n	Xanthan gum, calorie-free thickener
Vitaquick	VF	Sachet Tub	10g 100g 250g 1kg 6kg	* * * * *	n	Modified maize starch

Table 7.10 - Thickeners continued

Product	Manufac	Present	Volume/ Wt	ACBS Approv	Flavours	Comments

7

7

Section 8

General Data

Table 8.1 - Useful conversion factors

Parameter	Conversion factor
Weights and measures	$1oz = 28.35g = \sim 1$-2 tablespoons $16oz = 453.6g = 1lb = 0.45kg$ $5g = \sim 1$ teaspoon $1stone = 14lbs = 6.35kg$ $1kg = 2.2lbs = 1000g$ $1pt = 568mls$ $1l = 1000mls = 1.76pts$ $1g = 1ml = 1000mg$ $1ft = 0.31m = 30.48cm$
Energy from Macronutrients	$1kcal = 4.184KJ$ $1g$ Fat $= 9kcal = 38$ KJ $1g$ Alcohol $= 7kcal = 36$ KJ $1g$ Protein $= 4kcal = 17$ KJ $1g$ CHO $= 4kcal = 17$ KJ
Energy from IV Dextrose Solutions (Dextrose Monohydrate)	$1litre$ 5% (usual strength) $= 200$ kcal $1litre$ 25% $= 1000$ kcal $1litre$ 50% $= 2000$ kcal (500ml and 1l bags standard sizes)
Protein Equivalent	$1g$ AA $= 0.833g$ Protein
Nitrogen Equivalent	$1g$ Nitrogen $= 6.25g$ Protein
Sodium (Na)	$1*mmol\ Na^+ = 23mg\ Na^+ = 58.5mg NaCl$ $1g\ Na = 43.5mmol\ Na^+ = 2.5g\ NaCl$ $1g\ NaCl = 17.1mmol\ Na^+ = 393mg\ Na$ $1g\ NaHCO3 + 12mmol\ Na^+ = 327mg\ Na$ $1g\ MSG = 5.2mmol\ Na^+ = 120mg\ Na$ $1l$ normal saline $= 150mmol\ Na^+ = 3450mg\ Na$
Potassium (k)	$1\ mmol K^+ = 39mg K = 74.6mg\ Kcl$ $1g K^+ = 25.6mmol\ K^+ = 1.9g\ Kcl$
Vitamins	Vitamin D $1\mu g = 40$ IU Vitamin E $1mg = 1$ IU
mg $\longrightarrow$ mmol	$\dfrac{mg}{\text{atomic weight}}$
mmol $\longrightarrow$ mg	$mg = mmol\ x\ \text{atomic weight}$
Atomic weights	Sodium 23.0 Potassium 39.0 Calcium 40.0 Chloride 40.0 Chloride 35.4 Magnesium 24.3 Phosphorous 31.0 Sulphur 32.0

Source:McGinnity (1994) and BNF (1996).

*1mmol = atomic weight in mg

g	- grams	lb	- pound	kg	- kilogram
IU	- international units	oz	- ounce	pt	- pint
kcal	- kilocarlories	mg	- milligram	ml	- millilitre
l	- litre	μg	- microgram	KJ	- kilojules
mmol	- millimole				

Table 8.2 - Clinical blood biochemistry reference ranges

Parameter/units	Normal ranges	Comments
Sodium mmol/l	130 - 147	Hyponatraemia (low sodium) may indicate over-hydration (ie excessive fluid intake) or an insufficient dietary sodium intake. Diuretics may cause low sodium levels (as increased urine output increase sodium output). Hypernatraemia (high sodium) usually indicates dehydration or is indicative of reduced renal function
Potassium mmol/l	3.3 - 5.5	Often affected in renal failure or with diuretic treatment. Can partly reflect hydration status. In renal patients aim to keep levels <6. Both hyper and hypo-kalaemia can lead to cardiac dysfunction
Urea mmol/l	1.7-8.3 (20 - 30 normal for Renal patients)	Raised urea and sodium levels can indicate some renal impairment or dehydration. Low levels can indicate overhydration
Creatinine ummol/l	Males 60-125 Females 55-106	Raised levels can indicate renal impairment
Creatinine clearance ml/min	Males 95 - 140 Females 85 - 125	Used to measure Glomerular Filtration Rate (indicative of renal function). Raised levels can also indicate muscle protein degradation and negative Nitrogen balance
Phosphate mmol/l	0.8 - 1.6	Raised levels can indicate impaired renal function. Aim to keep levels <2.0 in renal patients. If low can affect adenosine triphosphate (ATP) synthesis (mainly seen in critically ill patients)
Albumin g/l	36 - 53	Poor short term indicator of protein mal-nutrition, since trauma and diseased states (such as liver and renal disease) and level of hydration can all affect level. Low albumin reduces oncotic pressure increasing risk of ascities/oedema
Total Protein g/l	66 - 87	Low levels may indicate protein malnutrition

8

Corrected Calcium (Ca) (for Albumin) mmol/l	2.20 - 2.26	Corrected for albumin of 42mmol/l. Albumin carries Ca round the body, therefore a low albumin may result in a low calcium level as well. Equation to calculate corrected Ca when albumin is < 40 = $$\text{measured calcium mmol/l} + \frac{(40 - \text{serum albumin})}{40}$$ Use corrected Ca or obtain ionised Ca levels at all times
Fasting glucose mmol/l	3.5 - 5.5	Fasting levels >7.8 indicates Diabetes
Glycosylated Haemoglobin (HbA1c) %	6.5 - 7.5% < 8% 8.1 - 9.6 > 10%	- Excellent Shows an average - Good blood glucose - Sub-optimal control over - Poor past 6 - 8 weeks
Haemaglobin (Hb) g/dl	M 13.0 - 18.0 F 11.5 - 16.5	More direct measure of Fe deficiency than haematocrit readings. Raised levels caused by dehydration/polycythemia. Decreased levels with haemorrhage/anaemia/protein-energy malnutrition. In renal pts, erythro-poeitin injections start when levels are < 8.0
Iron (Fe) umol/l	M 14 - 31 F 11 - 29	Raised values associated with Fe overload/haemolytic disorders/acute liver damage. Low levels occur with Fe deficiency anaemia/nephrosis infections
Total cholesterol mmol/l	3.4 - 5.2	A combination of lifestyle, genetics and diet will affect serum cholesterol levels. Serum cholesterol levels should be measured alongside other serum lipid parameters such as HDL, LDL and TG's for a more accurate lipid profile
High Density Lipoprotein (HDL) mmol/l	M 0.94-1.44 F 1.16-1.66	Transports excess cholesterol from cells to the liver for excretion in bile. High levels are therefore beneficial and are inversely related to heart disease.
Low Density Lipoprotein (LDL) mmol/l	< 4	Transports cholesterol from the liver to peripheral tissues. 60% of total cholesterol is found in LDL. LDL cholesterol is most closely associated with heart disease

8

Triglycerides (TG) mmol/l	0.8-1.9	Raised levels are associated with heart disease. Dietary TG are hydrolysed in the intestines and formed into micelles with bile salts and cholesterol.
Vitamins **A μmol/l** **B$_1$ nmol/l** **B$_2$ nmol/l** **B$_6$ nmol/l** **B$_{12}$ ng/l** **Ascorbate μmol/l** **D nmol/l** **E μmol/l**	0.7—1.7 > 40 total < 85.0 free < 21.3 > 178 160 - 925 34 - 68 24 - 111 10.2 - 39.0	Unlikely to routinely screen for all serum Vitamin levels in hospital since expensive and requires specialized equipment. Vit B12 injections are necessary for patients who have had a total gastrectomy, long term (if deficient in VitB12) due to loss of intrinsic factor.
pH	7.35 - 7.45	>7.45 = alkalosis <7.35 = acidosis
Bicarbonate mmol/l	22 - 32	Often altered in lung, kidney and liver disease. Affects acid base balance
Chloride mmol/l	95 - 107	Useful in determining the cause of acidosis
Bilirubin UMOL/L	0 - 19	Increased levels indicate jaundice
GAMMA GT u/l **ALT u/l** **Alkaline Phosphate ium/u/l** **CK u/l**	Males < 50 Females < 40 7 - 40 60 - 306 30 - 130 M <195 F < 170	Main cardiac enzyme measurement. Raised levels may indicate infarcted myocardial tissue, but may also reflect other damaged body tissue

Reference Ranges based on The Royal London and The Royal Hallamshire, Sheffield, Hospital Figures

Interpretation of Parameters, Ewald (1995)

3

Table 8.3 - Medical Shorthand

x/7	x days or x times a week	x	times
x/52	x weeks	x, ✓	dislikes, likes
x/12	x months	2222 or 55	resuscitation
∴	therefore	#	fracture
∵	because	<	less than
→	resulting in	>	greater than
1°	primary	△	diagnosis
2°	secondary	∧	abdomen
+ve	positive	∨	
-ve	negative	od	once a day
↑	increase	bd	twice a day
↓	decrease	tds	three times a day
↔	stable	qds	four times a day
1st	first	qqh	every four hours
2nd	second	prn	when required
2c	to see	ac	before food
♀	female	pc	after food
♂	male	om	in the morning
++	an excess of	on	at night

Submitted by Ms. Zoe Jenkins, SRD, St. James Hospital, Leeds

8

Medical abbreviations

A

a	at	am	morning
AA	Amino Acid	al	albumin
AAA	Abdominal Aortic Aneurysm	AML	acute myelogenous or myeloid leukaemia
AB	antibiotics	amt/s	amount/s
ac	before meals	AN	anorexia nervosa or antenatal
abdo	abdominal	ANF	antinuclear factor
ACBS	Advisory Committee on Borderline Substances	ADL	activities of daily living
		appt	appointment
ACEvits	Vitamins A,C & E	app	appropriate
AD	Alzheimer's Disease	AP	anterio-posterior
ADH	antidiuretic hormone	A-R	apical-radical (pulse)
AF	atrial fibrillation	ARDS	Acute Respiratory Distress Syndrome
AFB	acid-fast bacilli		
A/G	albumin globulin ratio	ARF	acute renal failure
AI	aortic insufficiency/incompetence	AS	alimentary system
		ASAP	as soon as possible
AID	artificial insemination (donor)	asp.n	aspiration
		ASCVD	arteriosclerotic cardio-vascular disease
AIDS	Acquired Immune Deficiency Syndrome	ASD	arterial septal defect
AKA	above knee amputation	ASHD	arteriosclerotic heart disease
ALS	amyotrophic lateral sclerosis	ASO	antistreptolysin O
		ATN	acute tubular necrosis
Amb	ambulant, ambulatory/ambulance	Aux	auxiliary
		AV	arteriovenous:artioventricular
A & E	Accident and Emergency	A + W	alive and well
ALL	acute lymphocytic leukaemia	AXR	abdominal x-ray

B

BaE	barium enema	BMTU	Bone Marrow Transplant Unit
BBB	bundle branch block		
BCAA	branched chain amino acids	BMTX	Bone Marrow Transplant
		BNF	British National Formulary
Bd/Bid	twice a day	BNO	bowels not open
BiD	brought in dead	BOR	bowels open regularly
Bil	bilirubin	BP	blood pressure
Bld	blood	BPH	benign prostatic hypertrophy
BKA	below the knee amputation	BS	blood sugar/bowel sounds/breath sounds
BM	blood sugar/glucose levels or bowel movement	BSS	blood sugar series
		BT	brain/breast tumour
		B/T	bedtime

BMI	body mass index	BUN	blood urea nitrogen
BMR	basal metabolic rate	Bx	biopsy

C

c̄	with	CML	chronic myeloid
c̲	without		leukaemia
C̲a	carcinoma,calcium	CMV	Cyto Megalo Virus
CABG	coronary artery bypass	CNA	cannot attend
	graft	CNS	central nervous system
Canc	cancelled	C/N	charge nurse
CAPD	continuous ambulatory	CRG	cardiac rehabilitation group
	peritoneal dialysis	CRP	C. Reactive Protein
CAT	computer assisted	C/O	complains of
	tomography	C/S	Church of Scotland
Cath.	Catholic or catheter	COAD	chronic obsturctive airway
CBC	complete blood count		disease
CCF	chronic cardiac failure	COLD	chronic obstructive lung disease
	failure/congestive	COPD	chronic obstructive pulmonary
	cardiac failure		disease
CCPD	continuous cyclical	CPK	creatinine phosphokinase
	peritoneal dialysis	CPR	cardiopulmonary resuscitation
CCU	coronary care unit	Creat/cr	creatinine
CDC	centres for disease	CRF	chronic renal failure
	control	CS	cardiovascular system
CDH	Children's Day Hospital	C + S	culture and sensitivity
C/E	Church of England	CSF	cerebrospinal fluid
CEA	carcinoembryonic	CSU	catheter specimen of urine
	antibody	C/T	continue treatment
cf	compared with	CT	computed tomography
CF	Cystic Fibrosis	CVA	cerebrovascular accident/
CFT	complement fixation test		costovertebral angle
CHD	coronary heart disease	CVD	cardio vascular disease
CHF	congestive heart failure	CVP	central venous pressure
CHO	carbohydrate	CVS	cardiovascular system
chol	cholesterol	Cx	cervix
CL	clubbing	CXR	chest x-ray
CLD	chronic liver disease	Cy	cyanosis
CMH	community and mental		
	health		

D

D,D	diagnosis	DNA	did not attend
D&C	dilation and curettage		(out-patients)
d/c	discharge, discontinue,	DOA	dead on arrival
	decrease	DOE	dyspnoea on exertion

8

DD,	differential diagnosis/	D/PP	differential count (WBC's)
	blood	D/Sal,	dextrose saline, dext/sal
diff	differential blood	D/S	diet sheet
DIC	disseminated intra-	dext	dextrose
	vascular coagulation	DTs	delirium tremens
DM	diabetes mellitus	DTR	deep tendon reflexes
D/N	day/night frequency	DU	duodenal ulcer
	(or urine)	DUB	dysfunctional uterine bleeding
DN	district nurse	D+V	diarrhoea and vomiting
DNS	Diabetes Nurse	DVT	deep vein thrombosis
	Specialist	D/W	discussed with
		DXT	deep x-ray therapy

E

EAA	essential amino acids	EMG	electromyography
ECG	electrocardiogram	EMI	elderly mentally infirm
EDC	expected date of	EMIT	enzyme immune assay
	confinement	ENG	electronystagmorgram
EDD	expected date of	EOM	extracelluar movement
	delivery	ERCP	endoscopic retrograde
ECT	electroconvulsive		cholangio-
	therapy		pancreatography
EEG	electroencephalogram	ESR	erythrocytesedi-
EFA	essential fatty acids		mentation rate
ENT	ears, nose and throat	EXP	expansion

F

FA	folic acid	FROM	full range of
FB	finger breadth/foreign		movement
	body	FTND	full term, normal
FBC	full blood count		delivery
FBS	fasting blood sugar	FTT	failure to thrive
FEV	forced expiratory	FUO	fever of unknown
	volume in 1 second		origin
FH	family history	Fx,#	fracture, also dose
FLP	fasting lipid profile		of radiation

G

g	gauge	GS	genital system
gast	gastrostomy	GSD	glycogen storage disease
GB	gall bladder	GT	gamma glytamyl transferase
GC	gonococci	gtt	guttac (drop)
GCS	Glasgow coma scale	GTT	Glucose Tolerance Test
GFR	glomerular filtration rate	GUM	genitourinary, medicine
GI,GIT	gastrointestinal tract	gyn	gynaecology
grav	gravid (pregnant)		

H

H	hypodermic	H & P	history and physical
Hb,Hgb	haemoglobin	HPC	history of present condition
HbA1c	glycosylated Hb		
Hct	haematocrit	hpf	high power field
HCVD	hypertensive cardi vascular disease	HO	House Officer
		HPI	history of present illness
HD	haemodialysis		
HDL	high density lipoprotein	HTVD	hypertensive vascular disease
HDU	high dependency unit		
HIV	Human Immuno-deficiency Virus	Hs,hs	bedtime
		HV	Health Visitor, Home Visit
HEENT	head, eyes, ears, nose and throat		

I

IBD	irritable bowel disease	I*O	intake and output
ICM	intracostal margin	IP	intraperitoneal
ICS	intercostal space	IPPB	intermittent positive pressure breathing
ICP	intracranial pressure		
ICU	intensive care unit	IPD	intermittent peritoneal dialysis
id	intradermal		
IDDM	insulin dependant diabetes mellitus	IRDM	insulin requiring diabetes mellitus
I & D	incision and drainage	ISQ	in status quo
ihd	intermittent haemodialysis	ITDM	insulin treated diabetes mellitus
IHD	ischaemic heart disease	iv	intravenous
		IVC	intravenous cholecystogram
im	intramuscular	IVN	IV nutrition
IMP	impression	IVP	intravenous pyelogram

J

J	jaundice	JVP	jugular venous pressure
jej	jejunostomy		

K

KO	keep open	KVO	keep vein open
KS	Kaposi's Sarcoma		

L

L	lymphadenopathy	LLL	left lower lobe (lung) or
L	left		left lower lid (eye)
LAT	lateral	LLQ	left lower quadrant (abdomen)
LBBB	left bundle branch block		
LBW	low birth weight	LMP	last menstrual period
LCFA	long chain fatty acid	LOW	loss of weight

8

LCT	long chain triglyceride	LP	lumbar puncture
LDL	low density lipoprotein	lpf	lower power field
LD	lethal dose	LSB	long stay bed (geriatric)
LDH	lactic dehydrogenase	LTX	liver transplant
LE	lupus erythematosus	LUQ	left upper quadrant (abdomen)
LFT	liver function test		
LIH	left inguinal hernia	LVF	left ventricular failure
LKS	liver, kidney, spleen	LVH	left ventricular hypertrophy

M

m^2	square meters body surface	meQ	mili-equivalent
M	murmur	MF	myocardial fibrosis, mycoses fungoides
MCFA	medium chain fatty acids	MI	myocardial infarction, mitral incompetence, mitral insufficiency
MCH	meancorpuscular haemoglobin	MIC	minimum inhibitory concentration
MCHC	mean corpuscular haemoglobin concentration	MMA	methyl malonic acidemia
		MND	Motor Neurone Disease
MCT	medium chain triglyceride	MS	Multiple Sclerosis, mitral stenosis
MCL	midclavicular line	MSU	midstream urine
MCV	mean corpuscular volume	MSUD	maple syrup urine disease
METS	metastases	MTA	mid-thigh amputation

N

N	normal	NIDDM	Non Insulin Dependent Diabetes Mellitus
NAD	nothing abnormal detected, no acute distress	#NOF	fractured neck of femur
		NPN	nonprotein nitrogen
NBM	nil by mouth	NS	nervous system (1-12 cranial nerves; T tone; P power; C co-ordination; S sensitive)
NEC	necrotising entero colitis		
NG	Nasogastric Tube Feed		
NHL	Non Hodgkin Lymphoma	NSR	normal sinus rhythm
NJ	Nasojejunal Tube Feed	N&V	nausea and vomiting

O

OA	on admission, osteoarthritis	OE	on examination
		OOB	out of bed
OB	occult blood	OPA	out-patient appointment
Ob-Gyn	obstetrics and gynaecology	OR	operating room
		Orthop-	orthopnea

8

OC	oral cholecystogram	OS	left eye
OD	right eye	OT	old tuberculin,
O/D	overdose		Occupational Therapy
od	every day/once a day	OU	both eyes
ODQ	on direct questioning	O	absent eg OBS=no bowel sounds

P

PA	propionic acidemia,	PMB	post menopausal bleeding
	posterio-anterior,	PMH	past medical history
	pernicious anaemia	PMI	point of maximum impulse
paed	paediatric	PMN	polymorphonuclear
PARA	number of pregnancies		leucocytes
para	paracetamol	PN	percussion note
PAT	paroxysmal atrial	PND	paroxysmal nocturnal
	tachycardia		dyspnoea
PBC	primary biliary cirrhosis	PNET	primitive neuro-
PBI	protein bound iodine		ectodermal tumour
PC	present condition,	PND	post-nasal drip
	after meals	PO	per os (by mouth)
PCP	pneumocystis carini	POD	paracetamol overdose
	pneumonia	POLY	polymorphonuclear
PCN	penicillin		leuccoyctes
PCV	packed cell volume	PPD	purified protein derivative
PE	physical examination,		(of tuberculin), packs per day
	pulmonary embolism	PPH	post-partum haemorrhage
PEC	pneumoencephalogram	PPN	peripheral parenteral nutrition
PEG	percutaneous endoscopic	PPT	partial prothrombin time
	gastrostomy	PR	plantar response, per rectum
PENG	Parenteral and Enteral	prn	when required
	Nutrition Group	pt	patient
PERRLA	pupils equal, round,	PT	prothrombin time,
	reactive to light and		Physiotherapy
	accommodation	PTA	prior to admission
PET	pre-eclamptic toxaemia	PTR	prothrombin ratio
PF	peak flow	PTT	partial thromboplastin time
PID	prolapsed intervertebral	PU	peptic ulcer
	disc, pelvic	PUO	pyrexia of unknown origin
	inflammatory disease	PV	per vagina
PKU	phenylketonuria	PVC	premature ventricular
PM	post mortem		contraction

Q

qd	every day	quid/qds	four times daily
qh	every hour	qod	every other day

R

R	right	RHD	rheumatic heart disease
RA	rheumatoid arthritis, right auricle/atrium	RLE	right lower extremity
		RLL	right lower lobe
rad	radical	RLQ	right lower quandrant
RBBB	right bundle branch block	RQ	respiratory quotient
		R/O	rule out
RBC	red blood count, red blood cell	ROS	review of symptoms
		RR	recovery room
RBS	random blood sugar	RS	respiratory system
RES	reticulo endothelial system	RSV	respiratory syncytial virus
		RTA	road traffic accident
RF	rheumatoid factor or respiratory failure	RTX	renal transplant
		RUQ	right upper quadrant
RFT	respiratory function tests	RVH	right ventricular hypertrophy

S

S	symptoms	SCID	severe combined immune deficiency
s	without		
S1	first heart sound	SDH	subdural haematoma
S2	second heart sound	SED	slow efficient dialysis
SA	sino-atrial	SGOT	serum glutamic oxaloacetic transaminase
SAH	subarachnoid haemorrhage		
		SGPT	serum glutamic pyruvic transaminase
SALT	Speech and Language Therapist	SH	social history
		sl	sublingual
SB	seen by	SLE	systemic lupus erythematosus
SBE	subacute bacterial endocarditis	SOA	swelling of ankle
		SOB	shortness of breath or stools for occult blood
sc	subcutaneous, subclavian		
		SOS	swelling of sacrum
SC	sclerosing cholangitis	SR	sedimentation rate
SCC	squamous cell carcinoma or spinal cord compression	SRD	state registered dietitian
		ss	saline solution
		STD	sexually transmitted disease
SCFA	short chain fatty acids		

T

T&A	tonsillectomy and adenoidectomy	TLC	total lung capacity or tender loving care
TAH	total abdominal hysterectomy	TM	tympanic membrane
		TOF	trachaeo-oesophageal fistula
TB	tuberculosis		

TCC	transitional cell carcinoma	TPI	treponema pallidum immobilization
TCI	to come in (out-patients)	TPN	total parenteral nutrition
		TPR	temp/pulse/respiration
TG	triglyceride	TPHI	treponema pallidum haemaglutination inhibition
TIA	transient ischaemic attack		
		TSH	thyroid stimulating hormone
TIBC	total iron binding capacity	TTA	to take away (medications and equipment)
tid or TDS	three times a day		
TITA	too ill to attend	TTO	to take out (to take home) transurethral (prostatic) resection
TKVO	to keep vein open	TURP	transurethral resection of prostate
		TX	treatment, therapy

U

UA	uric acid, urinalysis	URTI	upper respiratory tract infection
UC	ulcerative colitis		
U+E	urea and electrolytes	US	urinary system, ultrasound
UGI	upper GI series	UTI	urinary tract infection

V

v	very	VLCD	very low calorie diet
Vanc	vancomycin	VLDL	very low density lipoprotein
VLBW	very low birth weight	VMA	vanillymandelic acid

W

WCC	white cell count	wks	weeks
wd	ward	wt	weight
W/E	weekend		

X

xs	excess

Y

yrs	years	yds	yards

Z

ZF	zimmer frame

Main source submitted by Ms Zoe Jenkins, SRD, St James Hospital, Leeds and adapted by the author

8

Useful diet history/food abbreviations

A

alc/ETOH	Alcohol		

B

BE	Boiled egg	bp	Butter pat
Bix/bis/bic/bisc	Biscuits	BU	Build Up

C

cc or cr	Cream crackers	Cot	Cup of tea
CF	Cornflakes	C.P	Cheese portion
Choc	Chocolate	Chix	Chicken
coc	Cup of coffee		

D

DC	Double cream	Dig bi	Digestive biscuit
DM	Diabetic		

E

EM	Evening meal		

F

FE	Fried egg	FF	Full Fat
FCM	Full cream milk	FJ	Fruit Juice

G

g	grammes	Gfr	Grapefruit
GF	Gluten Free		

H

HP	High Protein	HF	High Fibre

I

IC	Ice cream		

J

Jkt	Jacket (Potato)		

K

Kcal	Calories	Kg	Kilograms

L

LFS	Low Fat Spread	Ib	Pounds
Low cal	Low Calorie		

M

Marg	Margarine	ml/s	millilitre/s
M/F	Meat/Fish	MP	Milk Puddings
MK	Main Kitchen	MW	Microwave

8

118

O

OJ	Orange Juice	oz	Ounces

P

PE	Poached egg	Pudd	Pudding
Pot	Potato	pb	Plain biscuits
Porr	Porridge	Pt.	Pint

R

R.K.	Rice Krispies	Rst/R	Roast

S

Sat	Saturated Fat	x SMP	Supplemented milk pudding
SE	Scrambled Egg		
SI	Slice	SMP	Skimmed milk powder
S/W or S'wich	Sandwich		
S.S.	Semi Skimmed	Supps	Supplements
ST	Silver Top	STF	Sweet Tinned Fruit
SF	Sugar Free		

T

T	Tinned	txd/liq	turmix/liquidized
Toms	Tomatoes		

V

Veg	Vegetables		

W

WBX	Weetabix	W/M	Wholemeal
W/E	Weekend		

Y

YP/Y.Pudd	Yorkshire pudding		

Meal times

BF/B'fast	Breakfast	PM	Afternoon
MM	Mid morning	EM	Evening meal
AM	Morning	S/Supp	Supper
L	Lunch	BB	Before bed
MA	Mid afternoon		

Submitted by Ms Zoe Jenkinson, SRD, St James, adapted by the author.

8

Table 8.4 - Food portion sizes and weights 'common foods'

(Approximate food portion sizes and weights per adult)

Food	Size and weight
Pasta, noodles, pasta shapes	1 very generous *cup uncooked 3oz (85g)
Rice	1/2 cup uncooked 2 - 3oz (55-85g)
Potatoes (medium)	3 - 4, according to size 8oz (225g)
White fish	6 - 8oz (170 - 225g)
Roast beef	6oz (170g)
Minced beef	4 - 6oz (110 - 170g)
Beef steak	6 - 8oz (170 - 225g)
Stewing steak	4 - 6oz (110 - 170g)
Chicken breast	6 - 8oz (170 - 225g)
Roast pork	8oz (225g)
Pork or gammon steak	6oz (170g)
Butter/margarine	0.3oz (10g) per serving on bread
Hard cheese eg cheddar	1 inch cub = 2.5cm cube 1oz (30g)
1 medium slice bread	1oz (25 - 30g)
1 medium egg	1.6oz (50g)
1 medium apple	2.5oz (75g)
1 packet of crisps	1oz (28g)
1 medium chocolate bar	1.8oz (54g)

8 Rounded up figures based on Davies and Dickerson (1991)

*cup=1 tea cup (drinking size cup) approximately 1/4 pint/5 fl oz/150ml

Table 8.5 - Nutritional composition of hospital food

Food	Energy (Kcal)	Protein (g)	Food	Energy (Kcal)	Protein (g)
Breakfast			**Evening meal**		
1 Slice bread and			Soup	50	0
butter	140	3	Main dish	200	20
Portion jam/			Vegetarian dish	120	5
marmalade	35	0	Potato/rice/pasta	150	3
Boiled egg	90	7	Vegetables	10	0
Fruit juice	65	0	2 slice sandwich	200	12
Cereal and milk	200	7	Meat/fish salad	120	12
1 teaspoon sugar	20	0	Cheese and biscuits	220	8
			Fruit	70	0
Lunch			Main dessert	200	2
Main meat/fish dish	200	20	Mousse/jelly	100	2
Vegetarian dish	170	5			
Potato/rice/pasta	150	3	**Miscellaneous**		
Vegetables	10	0	Tea/coffee and milk	15	0
Meat/fish salad	120	12	1 teaspoon sugar	20	0
Main pudding	220	3	Hot chocolate	60	2
Mousse/jelly	100	2	Bovril	10	0
Ice cream	140	2	Fizzy drinks		
Yoghurt	135	6	(not diet)	75	1
Custard/milk			Fruit	70	0
pudding	80	3	Chocolate bar	250	2
Cheese and biscuits	220	8	2 x plain biscuits	140	2
Fruit	70	0	2 x fancy biscuits	130	1
			Milk (glass)	120	6

NB Estimated values only, before recipy modification. The [1]DOH (1995) have now set out specific guidelines for the nutritional content of hospital food.

8

Table 8.6 - Nutritional composition of 'common foods'

Food	Portion size (g)	Energy (Kcal)	Protein (g)
Whole milk	100	65	3.3
Semi-skimmed	100	45	3.4
Skimmed	100	33	3.4
Yoghurt (natural)	150	84	7.7
(fruit)	150	135	6.2
1 egg	60	88	7.5
1 portion butter	10	90	0
1 slice hard cheese	40	165	10
Cream (double)	35	157	0.6
(single)	35	69	0.9
Ice-cream	75	146	2.7
1 slice bread	25	55	2.2
Cornflakes	30	110	3.0
2 cracker biscuits	15	70	1.0
Sweet biscuits	15	70	1.0
Chicken, roast	85	184	20.0
Beef, roast	85	133	25.0
Beefburger, fried	60	160	12.0
2 x sausages, grilled	90	240	12.0
Fish in batter	130	260	21.0
baked	120	120	22.0
Tuna fish in oil	95	275	22.0
Rice, boiled	165	200	3.6
Pasta, boiled	150	156	5.4
Potato boiled	150	120	2.0
roast	130	204	3.5
fried	130	330	5.0
Tomato, raw	60	20	0
Carrots, boiled	65	12	0.5
Apple	120	42	0
Banana	135	63	1.0
Orange	200	52	1.2
Sugar, 2 teaspoons	10	40	0
Chocolate	50	265	4.2
Crisps	25	140	2.0
Peanuts	30	171	7.3

Figures based on McCance and Widdowson (1995)

8

Table 8.7 - Energy content of alcoholic beverages

Beverage	Energy (kcal)
Beers, lager and cider	
Half pint (284ml/10 fl oz) of:	
Bitter	90
Brown ale	80
Light or mild ale	70
Ordinary strength lager	85
Low-alcohol lager	60
Dry cider	95
Sweet cider	110
Spirits	
1 pub measure (25ml/ 1/6 gill) of:	
Brandy, Whisky, Gin, Rum or Vodka	50
Wine	
An average glass (113ml/4fl oz) of:	
Dry, White or Red	75
Sweet White	100
Rose	85
Sherry	
1 Pub measure (50ml/1/3gill) of:	
Dry	55
Medium	60
Cream	70
Mixers, soft drinks	
Ordinary tonic	35
Low calorie tonic	0
Can of coke	130
Diet coke	0
Glass of orange juice	80

Rounded up figures based on McCance and Widdowson (1995)

8

Recommended alcohol intakes

Recommended maximum intakes - (DOH,1995)

- Women 2 - 3 units/day (14 - 21 units/week)
- Men 3 - 4 units/day (21 -28 units/week)

$\Rightarrow$ 8g Alcohol = 1 unit of alcohol = 56kcal

1 unit of Alcohol is equivalent to:

- 1/2 Pint ordinary beer, lager or cider
- a single pub measure of spirits* (whisky, gin, bacardi, vodka)
- a standard glass of wine (125 mls)
- a small glass of sherry
- a measure of vermouth or aperitif

*Gill measures in:

England/Wales	= ~1/6 gill
N. Ireland	= 1/4 gill
Scotland	= 1/5 or 1/4 gill

- In men 55 - 65% of body weight = water
- In women 45 - 55% of body weight = water
- Therefore women are more at risk of the harmful effects of alcohol than men because the absorbed alcohol is less dilute in womens' body fluids

Table 8.8 - Weaning Guide (for a normal, healthy baby)

Food group	Examples	Major nutrients	4-6 months	6-9 months	9-12 months	After 1 year	Additional information
Milk	Breast milk, infant formula, cow's milk (always full fat)	Energy and fat Protein, Calcium, Zinc, Iron, Vitamin A + B in breast and formula milks	Minimum 600ml breast or infant formula daily	500ml - 600ml breast milk, infant formula or follow-on formula daily	500ml - 600ml breast milk or infants daily milk	Minimum 350ml milk daily or 2 servings dairy products (eg yoghurt, cheese sauce)	If milk drinks are rejected, use alternatives (eg cheese and give water to drink Discourage large volumes of milk after 1 year (ie more than 600ml) as it will stop appetite for other foods. Discourage feeding from a bottle after 1 year.
Dairy produce and substitutes	Lassi, yoghurt*, fromage Frais*, cottage cheese Infant soya formula, tofu	As above	Cow's milk products can be used in weaning after 4 months (eg yoghurt custard, cheese sauce)	Also use any milk** to mix solids. Hard cheese (eg Cheddar) can be cubed or grated and used as 'finger food'		Whole milk can be used as a drink and soft cheeses included after 1 year. Lower fat milks can be used in cooking, but not as main drink.	

Table 8.8 - Weaning Guide (for a normal, healthy baby) continued

Food group	Major nutrients	Examples	4-6 months	6-9 months	9-12 months	After 1 year	Additional information
Starchy foods	Energy, Protein, thiamin, niacin, folic acid, vitamin B6, biotin, zinc. Calcium, iron (fortified cereal and bread) Non starch polysaccharide (Fibre)	Bread, rolls, pitta bread, chapatti, breakfast cereals, baby cereal, plain and savoury biscuits, noodles, spaghetti and other pasta, semolina, rice oats, millet, potato, yam, plantain	**Introduce after 4 months** Mix smooth cereal with milk; use low fibre cereals (eg rice based) Mash or puree starchy vegetables, rusks and baby rice	**2 - 3 servings daily** Start to introduce some wholemeal bread and cereals. Foods can be a more solid 'lumpier' texture. Begin to give 'finger' foods (eg toast) and bread sticks	**3 - 4 servings daily** Encourage wholemeal products; discourage foods with added sugar (biscuits, cakes etc) Starch foods can be of normal adult texture	**Minimum of 4 servings** At least one serving at each meal time Discourage high fat foods (crisps, savoury snacks and pastry)	Most baby and breakfast cereals are fortified with iron and B Vits Cereals and bread derived from wholemeals are a richer source of nutrients and fibre than refined cereals
Vegetables and fruit.	Vits A, C and Folate Non-Starch Polysaccharide use low-fibre	Leafy and green vegetables (cabbage, green beans, peas, broccoli, leeks) and salad. Fruit (apple, banana, peach, orange, melon). Fruit juices	**Introduce after 4 months** Mix smooth cereal with milk; banana, cereals (eg rice based) as 'finger foods' Mash or puree starchy veg	**2 servings daily** Raw soft fruit and veg (eg banana, melon, tomato) may be used as 'finger foods' Cooked veg and fruit can be a coarser, mashed texture	**3 - 4 servings daily.** Encourage lightly - cooked or raw fruit if veg are rejected. Chopped or 'finger food' texture is suitable. Unsweetened orange juice with meals especially if diet is meat free	**Minimum of 4 servings daily** Encourage unsweetened pies and stews. To improve iron absorption, give Vit C adult though some fibrous foods may be difficult (eg celery; radish)	Veg may be preferred raw (eg grated carrot, chopped tomato) or may need to be disguised in soups, pies and stews. To improve iron absorption, give Vit C fruits and veg with every meal

8

Table 8.8 - Weaning Guide (for a normal, healthy baby) continued

Food group	Examples	Major nutrients	4-6 months	6-9 months	9-12 months	After 1 year	Additional information
Meat and meat alternatives	Lean lamb, beef, pork, chicken, turkey, fish, fish fingers, egg, liver, kidney, sausages, burgers. Lentils, dhal, peas, beans, baked beans, gram, tofu and quorn	Energy and fat, protein, iron, zinc, B Vits (B12 animal foods only)	**Introduce after 4 months** Use soft-cooked meat/pulses. Add no salt or sugar or minimum quantities to food during or after cooking	**1 serving daily** Soft-cooked minced or pureed meat/ fish pulses. Chopped hard-cooked eggs can be used as a 'finger food'	**Minimum 1 serving daily from animal source or 2 from vegetable sources.** In a vegetarian diet use a mixture of different veg and starchy foods (macaroni cheese, dhal and rice)	**Minimum 1 serving daily or 2 from vegetable sources.** Encourage low fat meat and oily fish (sardine, herring, mackerel) Liver pate can be used after 1 year	Trim fat from meat Use little or no added fat when cooking foods which already contain fat such as meat
Occasional foods	Cakes, sweet biscuits, sweetened squash, sweetened desserts and milk drinks, ice cream, sugar, jam, honey etc, crisps, savoury snacks, fried and fatty foods	**None of these foods are necessary in the diet.** They may contain a lot of fat, energy, sugar or salt. Try not to use foods from this group every day	Choose low-sugar desserts; avoid high salt foods	Encourage savoury foods rather than sweet ones. Fruit juices are not necessary - try to restrict to meal times or alternatively offer water/milk	May use moderate amounts of butter, margarine. Small amounts of jam (if necessary) on bread Try to limit salty foods	Limit crisps and savoury snacks. Give bread or fruit if hungry between meals. Do not add sugar to drinks. Try to limit soft drinks to meal times and avoid fizzy drinks where possible	Encourage a pattern of three main meals each day. Discourage frequent snacking on fatty or sugary foods

Submitted by Anita Uprichard. Community SRD, North Tyneside General Hospital.

* These products should preferably be unsweetened varieties   **Includes breast milk, infant formula, follow-on formula and whole cow's milk
NB Breast milk, whenever possible, should always be encouraged in preference to formula milks as it is better designed for human babies and has several other health benefits over formula milk.

8

127

Table 8.9 - Water soluble vitamins

Vitamin/ RNI	Rich dietary sources	Deficiency diseases	Symptoms	Risk groups
C (Ascorbic acid) 40 - 60 mg	Citrus fruits, strawberries, nectarines, melons, vegetables, tomatoes, potatoes	Scurvy	Slow healing of wounds. Bleeding gums. Loose teeth	Pts who have undergone extensive, repeated surgery. Seriously ill pts with fever. Burns or tumour formation pts
B_1 (Thiamin) 0.8-1.1mg	Wheatgerm, yeast, liver, wholegrains, fish, poultry, beans and pork	Beriberi	Muscle paralysis Irritability Fatigue Mental confusion	Alcoholics Persons consuming refined diet
B_2 (Riboflavin) 1.1-1.3mg	Fortified breakfast cereals, meat, eggs, green leafy veg, offal pulses, dairy products	Aribo-flavinosis	Stomatitis (skin defects around the mouth and nose). Corneal Vascularization Glossitis	Women who are breast feeding or pregnant consuming an Insufficient quantity of dairy products. Pts with intestinal disease. Alcoholics
B_6 (Pyridoxine) 1.2-2.0mg	Fish. poultry, lean meats, nuts, pulses, wholegrain cereals, potatoes, bananas	Anaemia	Listlessness. Depression. Flaky skin around nose, mouth and eyes Poor body growth	Alcoholics Pregnant women Women taking the contraceptive pill
**B_{12} (Cyanocobalamin) 1.5-3.0µg	Offal, eggs, milk, oily fish, cheese, meat and other dairy products. Rich non meat sources include Barmen, Tastex, marmite, fortified soya milk and Ribena and fortified breakfast cereals	Pernicious Anaemia	Neurological defects	Vegans Gastrectomy pts
✝Folic acid (Folacin) 200-400 µg)	Green leafy veg, offal, milk products, meat, potatoes and fruit	Anaemia	Inflamed mucous membrane of GI tract	Pregnant women. Women taking contraceptive pill. Alcoholics. Pts with malabsorption disorders

Source: DOH (1991)

**Only when an intrinsic factor (produced in the stomach) and an extrinsic factor (contained in the vitamin) combine together can Vit B_{12} be utilised by the body. Which is why 'total gastrectomy' pts are likely to suffer from anaemia, unless they have regular Vit B_{12} injections.

✝Research has shown that folic acid can greatly reduce the chance of a baby being born with neural tube defects eg spina bifida by helping to make sure the babys spine develops properly. Women planning a pregnancy are advised to take a 400 mcg folic acid supplement as soon as contraception is discontinued to the twelfth week of pregnancy. Rich dietary sources of folic acid should also be encouraged.

NB Other water soluble vitamins include biotin, niacin and pantothenic acid.

Table 8.10 - Fat soluble vitamins

Vitamin/ RNI	Rich dietary sources	Deficiency diseases	Symptoms	Risk groups
✞A (Retinol) 600-1200 μg	Liver, eggs, oranges, yellow and green fruits and veg, milk and dairy products, fatty fish	Xeroph-thalmia (night blindness)	Poor dark adaptation Corneal sores Stunted growth, fatigue	Patients using laxatives Patients with poor fat digestion, eg Cystic fibrosis and pancreatitis patients
D None due to action of sunlight on skin, RNI 65 yrs+ 5μg	Oily fish, egg yolks, offal, fortified margarine and spreads, full fat milk and cheese	Rickets	Weak/soft bones (Osteo-malacia) Deformation of bones and teeth Calcium loss from bones	Elderly confined indoors Dark skinned children Patients with disturbed fat digestion
E (Toco-pherals) 10mg	Veg oils, green veg, wheatgerm, offal, eggs, cereals, nuts	Anaemia Muscular degener-ation (Myopathy) Reproductive failure Nerve damage	Instability of membrane structures Changes in connective tissue	Patients with poor fat digestion
K 1μg/kg body weight	Green leafy veg, liver, oils, potatoes, fruits, dairy products	Reduced Haemolysis (↓blood clotting factor)	Delayed blood coagulation	New born babies Patients on antibiotics or medication which affects the intestinal flora Patients on 'blood thinning' medications

Source: DOH (1991)

✞An excess of Vit A (more than 3300μg/day) during pregnancy has been asociated with an increased incidence of birth defects. As a precautionary measure therefore women in the UK who are, or might become pregnant, are advised not to take Vit A containing supplements unless otherwise advised by a doctor or antnatal clinic.

8

Table 8.11 - Minerals

Mineral/RNI	Rich dietary sources	Functions
Calcium 20mmol (0.2mmol/mg body weight)	Milk, dairy products and fish. Rich non dairy sources include fortified soya milks, fortified bread, spring cabbage, broccoli, apricots, raisins, almonds and cashew nuts	Strong bones, teeth, muscle tissue, regulated heart beat, muscle action and nerve function, blood clotting
Chromium 0.5-1.0µmol **Safe Intake	Brewers yeast, meat, wholegrains, legumes and nuts	Glucose metabolism (energy), increase effectiveness of insulin
Copper 16-20µmol	Oysters, nuts, offal, legumes	Formation of red blood cells, bone growth growth and health, works with Vit C to form elastin
Iodine 1.0 - 1.2 µmol	Seafoods, sea salt, milk and dairy products	Component of hormone thyroxine which controls metabolism
✝Iron 170-260µmol	Lean meat, offal and fish. Rich non meat sources include eggs, pulses, nuts and seeds, dried fruit, whole grain foods and wheatgerm, dark green veg and fortified breakfast cereals	Haemoglobin formation, improves blood quality, increases resistance to stress and disease
Magnesium 12-14mmol/day	Nuts, green veg, wholegrains	Acid/alkaline balance, important in metabolism of carbohydrates, minerals and sugar
Manganese 30-60µmol	Tea, nuts, wholegrains, fruits and veg	Enzyme activations, carbohydrate and fat productions, sex hormone production, skeletal development
Phosphorus 25mmol/day (0.3mmol/kg body weight)	Fish, meat, poultry, eggs, cereal and cereal products	Bone development, important in protein, fat and carbohydrate utilization
Potassium 50-100 mmol (1.0mmol/kg body weight)	Meat, veg, fruit, beans, dried peas, potatoes, fish, pork	Fluid balance, controls activity of heart muscle, nervous system, kidneys
Selenium 0.8-0.9µmol	Seafood, offal, lean meats, eggs, wholegrains	Protects body tissues against oxidative radiation, pollution and normal metabolic processing
Zinc 110-145µmol	Lean meats, liver, eggs, cheese, seafood,	Involved in digestion and metabolism, important in the development of reproductive system, aids in healing

Source: DOH (1991).

**Safe Intake:-A term used where there is currently insufficient information to estimate requirements. It is a level judged to be adequate for almost everyone's needs while not large enough to cause undesirable effects.

8

✢Upper level applies for women with high menstrual losses where the most practical way of meeting their iron requirements is to take iron supplements.

NB Other minerals include chloride, sodium, cobolt, fluoride and molyodenum.

Table 8.12 - Chemical elements and symbols

A		**H**		**P**	
Ag	Silver	H	Hydrogen	P	Phosphorus
Al	Aluminium	He	Helium	Pb	Lead
As	Arsenic	Hg	Mercury	Pt	Platinum
Au	Gold				
		I		**R**	
B		I	Iodine	Ra	Radium
B	Boron				
Ba	Barium	**K**		**S**	
Be	Beryllium	K	Potassium	S	Sulphur
Bi	Bismuth			Se	Selenium
Br	Bromine	**L**		Si	Silicon
		Li	Lithium	Sn	Tin
C				Sr	Strontium
C	Carbon	**M**			
Ca	Calcium	Mg	Magnesium	**T**	
Cd	Cadmium	Mn	Manganese	Ti	Titanium
Cl	Chlorine	Mo	Molybdenum	Tl	Thallium
Co	Cobalt			Tu	Tungsten
Cr	Chromium	**N**			
Cu	Copper	N	Nitrogen	**U**	
		Na	Sodium	U	Uranium
F		Ni	Nickel		
F	Fluorine			**V**	
Fe	Iron	**O**		V	Vanadium
		O	Oxygen		
G				**Z**	
Ga	Gallium			Zn	Zinc

Submitted by Ms Zoe Jenkins, SRD, St James Hospital, Leeds

8

Table 8.13 - A guide to religious influences on diet

Food	Jewish	Muslim	Hindu	Sikh	Buddhist	Rastafarian	Seventh Day Adventist
Eggs	no blood spots	✓	some	✓	some	some	most
Milk/ Yoghurt	✓	some	some	✓	✓	some	most
Cheese	not with rennet	not with rennet	not with rennet	some	✓	some	most
Pork	x	x	rarely	rarely	some	x	x
Beef	Kosher	Halal	x	x	some	some	some
Lamb	Kosher	Halal	some	✓	some	some	some
Chicken	Kosher	Halal	some	some	some	some	some
Fish	with scales, fins and backbone	with fins and scales	with fins and scales	some	some	with fins and scales	with fins and scales
Shellfish	x	some	some	some	x	x	x
Animal fats	Kosher	Halal	some	some	some	some	x
Alcohol	✓	x	x	✓	x	not usually wine	x
Cocoa/ coffee/tea	✓	✓	✓	✓	✓	x	De-caffeinated are suitable

			-	-	-	Processed, preserved and tinned foods often avoided. Most only eat *Ital* foods (those in whole and natural state). Fruits of the vine including sultanas, grapes and currants may be avoided
Fasting	Yom Kippur - Day of atonement (1 day) No food or liquids for 25 hours	Ramadan (1 month - daylight hours). Fasting involves abstinence from any food or liquids during daylight hours	3 fast days in a year. Devout Hindus may fast on 1 - 2 days per week	-	-	-
Other comments	Kosher means that the food is fit to eat by Jewish people, eg meat has been slaughtered in the prescribed manner by a Kosher butcher. Milk and dairy products are not consumed with a meal containing meat. Following a 'meat' meal a gap of up to 3 hours must be left before dairy products can be consumed	Halal means that the meal contains meat prepared according to Islamic law, ie the animal must bleed to death whilst prayers are said over it. Observant Muslims will also avoid foods which may contain 'haram' (forbidden) foods. So they may not eat foods with unspecified animal fat because it may contain pork, eg gelatin	Certain foods are taken during prayers	Some Sikhs may be vegetarian	Some Buddhists may not be vegetarian	

Source: Wet *et al* (1995), reproduced with kind permission.

some = eaten by some people   most = eaten by most people   ✓ food acceptable   x food not acceptable

8

133

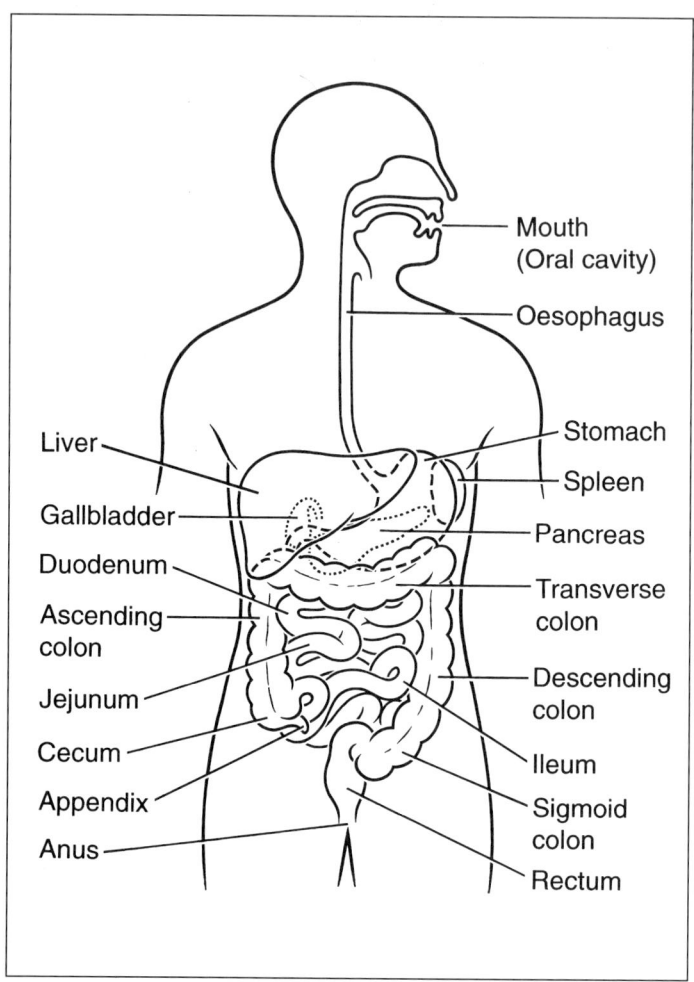

Fig 8.1 - Anatomy of the GI tract

Source: Tortora (1996)

8

Table 8.14 - Nutrition absorption sites in the GI tract

GI Site	Nutrient(s) absorbed	Comments
Stomach	None	B_{12} Intrinsic factor present
Duodenum	Minerals, Monosaccharides, Disaccharides, fatty acids, Vit A and D, water and sodium	Most minerals are absorbed at this point Only small amounts of remaining nutrients (except for water and sodium) absorbed here
Jejenum	Water, sodium, mono and disaccharides, Vit A and D, fatty acids, amino acids and simple peptides, water soluble vitamins	Most water soluble vits, amino acids and simple peptides, dissacharides and water/sodium absorbed at this point
Ileum	Bile salts, Vit B_{12}, water/ sodium, amino acids and simple peptides, water soluble vits	All Vit B_{12} absorbed and most of bile salts
Colon	Water/sodium, Vit K and potassium	Vit K formed by bacterial action

Source: Whitney *et al* (1991)

Table 8.15 - Amino acids in man

*Essential amino acids	Non-essential amino acids	Branched chain amino acids
Iso Leucine	Alanine	Leucine
Leucine	Arginine	Isoleucine
Lysine	Aspartic acid	Valine
Methionine	Cystine	
Phenylalanine	Glutamic acid	
Valine	Glycine	
Threonine	Histidine	
Tryptophan	Hydroxy proline	
	Proline	
	Serine	
	Tyrosine	
	Ornithine	

Source: Thomas B (1994)

*Essential amino acids cannot be synthesised by man, therefore they have to be obtained through dietary sources.

Table 8.16 - Normal fluid balance (adults)

In	ml	Out	ml
Oral fluids	1500	Faeces	200
Water from solid food	600	Insensible losses -	
Water from oxidation		lungs	400
(20ml/240J)	300	skin	400
		Sweat (temperate	
		climate)	200
		Urine	1200
Total	2400	Total	2400

Source: Entwistle (1992)

8

Table 8.17 - Dietetic and nutrition internet sites

The British Dietetic Association
http://www.bda.uk.com

The American Dietetic Association
http://www.eatright.org/

Dietetics Online
http://www.dietetics.com/

The Royal Bournemouth Hospital Nutrition & Dietetic
Department
http://www.rbch-tr.swest.nhs.uk/

The 'Virtual' Nutrition Centre
http://www-sci.lib.uci.edu/~martindale/

Nutrition and Health
http://www.medlib.arizona.educ/nutrition.html

Nutrition and Diseases
http://www.medlib.arizona.edu/educ/nu-disea.htm

Food and Nutrition Information Centre
http://www.nalusda.gov/fnic/

International Food Information Council
http://ificinfo.health.org/info-con.htm

World Health Organisation
http://www.who.ch/

Hospital Web
http://neuro-www.mgh.harvard.edu/hospitalweb.nclk

The Visible Human Project
http://www.nlm.nih.gov/research/visible/visible_human.html

Pharmaceutical Information Network
http://pharminfo.com/pin_hp.html

The British Medical Journal
http://www.bmj.com/bmj/

SHS Neocate
http://www.connect.org.uk/shs/neocate

Source: Compiled by the author

8

Table 8.18 - UK manufacturers' addresses for clinical nutrition products

Manufacturer	Address
Baxter Healthcare Ltd	Wallingford Rd, Compton, Newbury, Berkshire RG16 OQW T: (01635) 200000
(Mead Johnson) Bristol-Myers Squibb Pharmaceuticals	141-149 Staines Rd, Hounslow, Middlesex TW3 3JB T: (0181) 572 7422
Clintec Nutrition Ltd	Shaftesbury Court, 18 Chalvey Park, Slough, Berkshire SL1 2HT T: (01753) 550 800
Cow and Gate Nutricia Ltd	Newmarket Avenue, Whitehorse Business Park, Trowbridge, Wilts BA14 OXQ T: (01225) 768381
Everfresh Natural Foods	Gatehouse Close, Aylesbury, Bucks HP19 3DE T: (01296) 25333
Flexicare Medical Ltd	East Quay, Bridgewater, Somerset T: (01278) 458451
Foodwatch Health Products Ltd	Pollards Yard, Wood Street, Taunton, Somerset TA1 1UP T: (01823) 325023
Fresenius Ltd	6/8 Christleton Court, Stuart Rd, Manor Park, Runcorn, Cheshire WA7 1ST T: (01928) 579333
General Dietary Ltd	PO Box 38, Kingston Upon Thames Surrey KT2 7UP T: (0181) 336 2323
Gluten Free Foods Ltd	PO Box 178, Stanmore, Middlesex, HA7 4XN T: (0181) 954 73 48
Heinz H J Co Ltd	Haynes Park, Haynes, Middlesex UB4 8AL T: (0181) 848 2386
Hypoguard (UK) Ltd	Dock Lane, Melton, Woodbridge, Suffolk IP12 1PE T: (01394) 387333

8

Jacobs Bakery Ltd	Suttons Business Park, Earley, Reading, RG 6 1AZ T: (01734) 492000
Kimal Scientific Poducts Ltd	Arundel Rd, Uxbridge, Middlesex, UB8 2SA T: (01895) 270 951
(Boots) Knoll Ltd	9 Castle Quay, Castle Bouvlevard Nottingham, NG7 1FW T: (0115) 924 0909
Life and Light Eggs	St. Giles Foods, Unit 5, Church Estate, Slade Green Rd, Slade Green, Kent DA8 2JA T: (01322) 337711
Liposome Co Ltd	3 Shortlands, Hammersmith International Centre, London W6 8EH T: (0181) 3240058
Milupa Ltd	Uxbridge Rd, Hillingdon, Uxbridge Middlesex, UB10 ONE T: (0181) 573 9966
Monmouth Pharmaceutical Ltd	3(D1) Huxley Rd, Surrey Research Park, Guildford, Surrey, GU2 5RE T: (01483) 65299
Nestle Clinical Nutrition	Trinity Court, Church Street Rickmansworth, Hertfordshire, WD3 1LD T: (01923) 897772 F: (01923) 897603
Nestle UK Ltd	St. Georges House, Croydon Surrey, CR9 1NR T: (0181) 686 3333
Norgine Ltd	Chaplin House, Widewater Place, Moorhall Rd, Harefield, Middlesex, UB9 6NS T: (01895) 826600
Nova Nordisk Pharmaceuticals Ltd	Broadfield Park, Brighton Rd, Pease Pottage, Crawley, West Sussex, RH11 9RT T: (01293) 613555

8

Novartis Nutrition UK Ltd	Station Road, Kings Langley Herfordshire, WD4 8LJ T: (01923) 266122
Nutricia Clinical Care Ltd	White Horse Business Park, Trowbridge, Wiltshire BA14 0XQ T: (01225) 711677
Panpharma Ltd	Panpharma House, Repton Place, White Lion Rd, Little Chalfont, Amersham, Bucks, HP7 9LP T: (01494) 766866
Pharmacia and Upjohn Ltd	Milton Keynes Energy Park Davey Avenue, Knowlhill, Milton Keynes, Bucks MK5 8PH T: (01908) 661101
Robinson Healthcare	Hipper House, Chesterfield, S40 1YP T: (01246) 220022
Roche Products Ltd	PO Box 8, Welwyn Garden City, Herts AL7 3AY T: (01707) 366000
Ross Products Division	Abbott Laboratories Ltd, Abbott House, Nolden Road, Maidenhead, Berkshire SL6 4XE T: (01628) 773355
Salt and Sons Ltd	Saltair House, Lord St, Nechells, Birmingham, B7 4DS T: (0121) 359 5123
Scientific Hospital Supplies (UK) Ltd	100 Wavertree Boulevard, Wavertree Technology Park, Liverpool L7 9PT T: (0151) 228 1992
Smithkline Beecham Consumer	11 Stroke Poges Lane, Slough, Berkshire, SL1 3NW T: (01753) 533433 F: (01753) 502007
Sunderland Health Ltd	Unit 5, Rivermead, Pipers Way Thatcham, Berks RG13 4TP T: (01635) 874488

Unigreg Ltd	Enterprise House, 181/191 Garth Rd, Morden, Surrey, SM4 4LL T: (0181) 330 1412 Nutrition Department F: (0181) 337 4796 Unigreg Nutrition Helpline Freephone 0800 373698 Email: Admin@Unigreg.co.uk
Vitaflow Ltd	6 Moss St, Paisley, PA1 1BJ T: (01800) 515174
Wyeth Laboratories	Huntercombe Lane South Maidenhead, Berks SL6 OPH T: (01628) 604377

Source: Data Compiled from the BNF (95) by the author

Table 8.19 - Dietetic addresses - other

Society	Address
British Association of Parenteral and Enteral Nutrition	PO Box 922, Maidenhead, Berkshire, SL6 4SH
British Diabetic Association	10 Queen Anne St, London, W1M OBD T: 0171 323 1531 F: 0171 637 3644
British Dietetic Association	7th Floor, Elizabeth House 22 Suffolk St, Queensway, Birmingham, B1 1LS T: 0121 643 5483 F: 0121 633 4399 E: bda@dial.pipex.com
Coeliac Society	PO Box 220, High Wycombe, Bucks HP11 2HY T: 01494 437278
Council for Professions supplementary to Medicine	Park House, 184 Kennington Park Rd, London SE11 4BU T: 0171 582 0866
Eating Disorders Association	Sackville Place, 44 Magdalen St, Norwich, Norfolk NR3 1JU T: 01603 619090 F: 01603 664915
The National Centre for Clinical Audit	BMA House, Tavistock Sq London, WC1H 9JB T: 0171 383 6451 F: 0171 383 6373 E: NCCA@kcl.ac.uk
The Vegan Society	7 Battle Rd, St Leonards-on-Sea, East Sussex TN37 7AA
The Vegetarian Society	Parkdale, Durham Rd, Altrincham, Cheshire WA14 4QG

Source: Compiled by the author

References and further reading

British National Formulary (Sept 1996)
British Medical Association and the Royal Pharmaceutical Society of Great Britain

Davies J; Dickerson J (1991)
Nutrient Content of Food Portions, The Royal Society of Chemistry, Cambridge

Department of Health (1991)
Dietary Reference Values for Food Energy and Nutrients For The United Kingdom, Soc Subj 41. HMSO, London

[1]Department of Health (1995)
Nutrition guidelines for hospital catering: The Health of the Nation

[2]Department of Health (1995)
Sensible Drinking: Report of an Interdepartmental Working Group

Entwistle I R (1992)
Exacta Medica: Reference Tables and Data For The Medical and Nursing Professions, Churchill Livingstone

Ewald G (1995)
Manual of Medical Therapeutics, Little Brown

Facinoli S L (1996)
A Nutritionist Field Guide to Cyberspace, Journal of Nutrition Education 28 (1) pp26-32

Holland B; Welch A A; Unwin I D; Buss D H; Paul A A; Southgate D A T (1991)
McCance and Widdowson's The Composition of Foods, 5th ed. The Royal Society of Chemistry, Cambridge

Kiley R (1996)
Medical Information on the Internet; A guide for Health Professionals, Churchill Livingstome

McCance and Widdowson (1995)
The composition of foods. Royal Society of Chemistry, Ministery of Agriculture, Fisheries and Food, 5th edition

8

McGinnity (1994)
Dietitian's Pocket Book, Produced in house by Curtin University of Technology, Perth W. Australia

Micklewright A; Todorovic V (1989)
A Pocket Guide to Clinical Nutrition, Parenteral Enteral Nutrition Group of The British Dietetic Association

Naythons M; Catsimatides A (1995)
The Internet, Health Fitness and Medicine Golden Directory, Osborne McGraihill

Passmore R, Eastwood M A, Davidson and Passmore (1986)
Human Nutrition and Dietetics, 8th Edition, Churchill Livingstone

Thomas B (1994)
Manual of Dietetic Practice, 2nd edition. Blackwell Scientific Publications

Tortora G J, Geraro J, Anagnostakos, Nicholas P, Grabowski, Reynos (1996)
Principles of Anatomy and Physiology, Addison Wesley Longman

Wet M, Jean-Marie, Nelson J, Todd S and Zaidner T (1995)
Food and Culture, Community Nutrition Group of the British Dietetic Association

Whitney E N, Cataldo C B, Rolfes (1991)
Understanding Normal and Clinical Nutrition, 3rd Edition, West Publishing Co, USA

8

Notes

8